FITTING PANDEMIC SOLUTIONS TO SCALE

AN INVESTMENT ROAD MAP FOR MORE EQUITABLE, EFFECTIVE, AND AGILE PANDEMIC PREVENTION, PREPAREDNESS, AND RESPONSE

APRIL 2026

ASIAN DEVELOPMENT BANK

ADB

6 ADB Avenue, Mandaluyong City, 1550 Metro Manila, Philippines
Tel +63 2 8632 4444; Fax +63 2 8636 2444
www.adb.org

ISBN 978-92-9277-782-1 (print); 978-92-9277-783-8 (PDF); 978-92-9277-784-5 (ebook)
Publication Stock No. TCS260159-2
DOI: http://dx.doi.org/10.22617/TCS260159-2

Notes:
In this publication, “$” refers to United States dollars.
ADB recognizes “China” as the People’s Republic of China and “Korea” as the Republic of Korea.

Cover design by Cleone Baradas.

CONTENTS

TABLE, FIGURES, AND BOXES

TABLE

FIGURES

BOXES

FOREWORDS

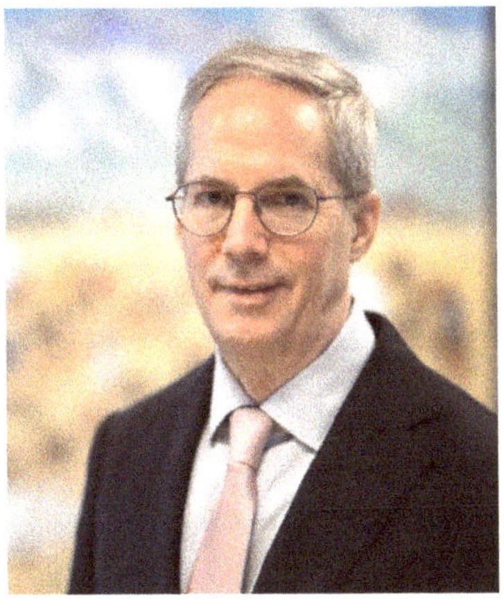

It has been 6 years since the outbreak of the coronavirus disease (COVID-19) pandemic. With the emergency period well behind us, it is essential that we prioritize the lessons learned from this extraordinary health, humanitarian, and economic crisis. Yet, calls for better pandemic preparedness struggle for attention in a global health landscape that is facing a growing array of challenges. Economic and geopolitical instability coupled with reduced development aid and competing investment priorities have placed developing member countries under fiscal pressure, putting unprecedented strains on health financing. At the same time, many countries in Asia and the Pacific are still grappling with the long tail of COVID-19 in the form of health and fiscal burdens. Against this backdrop, governments can no longer afford to think about health as separate from the broader economic, social, and national security systems in which it operates. Similarly, policymakers are increasingly looking to regional cooperation and regional resilience as necessary strategies to meet these increasingly complex, interconnected challenges.

This publication, *Fitting Pandemic Solutions to Scale: An Investment Road Map for More Equitable, Effective, and Agile Pandemic Prevention, Preparedness, and Response*, presents an evidence-driven road map to strengthen pandemic prevention, preparedness, and response in a regional context. Drawing on the insights of government leaders, researchers, industry experts, and multilateral partners who convened at the Asian Development Bank's (ADB) Symposium on Multilateral Financing for Pandemic Preparedness and Response, held in July 2025, the report offers three key lessons that are vital for Asia and the Pacific.

First, strong and resilient health systems must be the foundation of preparedness. COVID-19 revealed that emergency response capacities cannot stand apart from routine systems. Investments in primary health care, surveillance, laboratories, supply chains, and epidemiologic training generate benefits that extend far beyond emergencies, strengthening countries' ability to absorb, adapt, and rapidly respond. This reinforces a core message from the publication: preparedness and universal health coverage are mutually reinforcing, not competing, priorities.

Second, equitable access to vaccines, therapeutics, and diagnostics is both a moral imperative and a regional public good. During the pandemic, fragmented procurement, regulatory bottlenecks, and concentrated manufacturing capacity limited access for many developing member countries. Asia and the Pacific must avoid a repeat of these inequities. The publication highlights the need for a regionally integrated ecosystem for research and development, manufacturing, regulatory convergence, and collaborative procurement, supported by strong national regulators and coordinated regional platforms.

Third, financing must be predictable, agile, and aligned with country systems. COVID-19 demonstrated that delays in financing translate directly into lost lives and deeper economic disruption. The report calls for day-zero financing mechanisms, improved public financial management systems, and innovative financing approaches—including blended finance and coordinated surge financing. Preparedness financing must transition from reactive, fragmented support to sustained investments embedded in national budgets and regional frameworks.

These lessons align strongly with the direction set in ADB's Strategy 2030 Midterm Review, which places renewed emphasis on regional cooperation and integration, the delivery of regional public goods, and the strengthening of social and institutional resilience. In particular,

- Regional public goods—such as shared surveillance platforms, pooled procurement mechanisms, and coordinated manufacturing capacity—are central to preventing the next pandemic;
- Regional cooperation and integration are essential for harmonizing regulatory standards, strengthening cross-border data systems, and building supply-chain resilience; and
- Social and institutional resilience, as reinforced in the Midterm Review, requires embedding health emergency preparedness into broader development planning, fiscal frameworks, and cross-sector investments.

ADB is committed to supporting this transformation, drawing on our own experience from the past crisis. ADB's Asia Pacific Vaccine Access Facility, which helped to deliver over 675 million COVID-19 vaccine doses, showing that multilateral institutions can accelerate effective responses when financing, technical expertise, and partnerships are aligned. But too often they are not.

Looking ahead, we must ensure that preparedness becomes a permanent feature of development planning, not a temporary reaction to crisis. With climate change, demographic pressures, and rapid urbanization amplifying health risks, the next outbreak is a matter of when, not if. The guidance in this publication offers governments, development institutions, and the private sector a coherent investment pathway—one that strengthens resilience today and safeguards prosperity for the future.

I hope that this publication helps catalyze the collective action needed to build a more secure, equitable, and agile Asia and the Pacific. By investing strategically and collaboratively now, we can ensure that our region is far better prepared for the challenges that lie ahead.

Scott Morris
Vice-President (East and Southeast Asia, and the Pacific)
Asian Development Bank

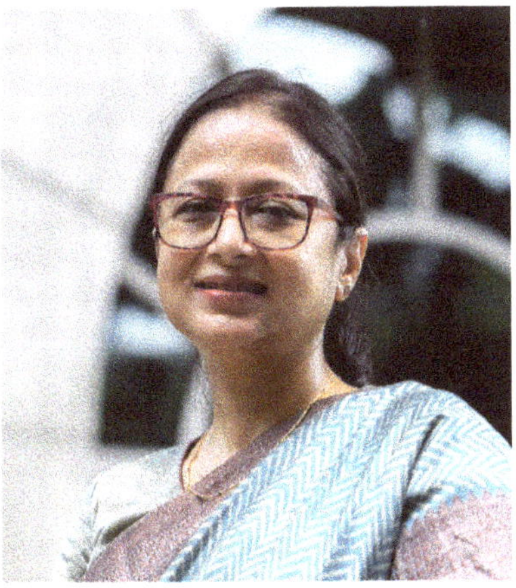

Evidence shows that the frequency of pandemics is on the rise. In Asia and the Pacific, population growth, urbanization, and climate shocks are exacerbating the spread of infectious diseases —elevating health security risks and intensifying the need for robust public health infrastructure. In the wake of COVID-19, these evolving risks offer an opportunity for significant reform. This includes rethinking the ways in which the region builds resilience against future outbreaks.

Yet, while health systems are the first line of defense during pandemics, critical funding shortfalls remain. Countries need more sustainable financing for pandemic preparedness and response. This requires governments to increase domestic resource mobilization and to better track pandemic spending. It also requires multilateral partners to establish sustained, predictable financing mechanisms aimed at building up core pandemic-related capacities—including strengthening universal health coverage and primary health care as the backbone of health systems. The pandemic demonstrated that it is also vital to scale investments in regional manufacturing and procurement of vaccines, therapeutics, and diagnostics. Sustainable financing and procurement should be underpinned by strategic coordination across the region and robust governance frameworks, with strong country ownership and accountability.

ADB is already supporting countries in Asia and the Pacific to address some of these priority actions. Regional initiatives such as the Asia Diagnostics, Vaccines, and Therapeutics Network to Counter Epidemics and the Ending Complex and Challenging Infectious and Tropical Diseases focus on increasing regional access to vaccines and reducing the frequency and impact of climate-sensitive diseases. These approaches for shared learning and collective action mirror recommendations brought to the fore during ADB's first Symposium on Multilateral Financing for Pandemic Preparedness and Response. We hope that the findings presented in this report help to unlock even more resources and accelerate high-impact integrated actions for stronger, more resilient health systems in Asia and the Pacific.

Fatima Yasmin
Vice-President (Sectors and Themes)
Asian Development Bank

ACKNOWLEDGMENTS

This report draws on the generosity and expertise of a long cast of contributors, most of whom traveled to Manila to participate in the Inclusive, Sustainable, Prosperous, and Resilient (INSPIRE) Health Forum of the Asian Development Bank (ADB), held on 7–11 July 2025.

The editors are grateful to the strategic guidance provided by Ayako Inagaki, senior director, Human and Social Development Sector Office, ADB; and David Oldfield, senior advisor to the Vice-President.

The writing team acknowledges the invaluable contributions of the SD3-HSD Health Practice Team and the VPR2 Office Team, without whose support the Symposium on Multilateral Financing for Pandemic Preparedness and Response in July 2025 could not have been held.

Thanks also go to Karmela Dua for leading the publication process, Toby Miller and Joy Quitazol-Gonzalez for copy editing and proofreading, Cleone Baradas for cover design, and Alvin Tubio for publication layout, and the entire DOCK team.

ADB Editors:
Nansubuga Nagadya Isdahl, consultant; **Benjamin Coghlan**, consultant; and **Jae Kyoun Kim**, health specialist.

Authors:
Ruchir Agarwal, director of the Raj Center on Indian Economic Policies, School of International and Public Affairs, Columbia University; **Dinesh Arora**, principal health specialist, ADB; **Eduardo Banzon**, director of Health, ADB; **Helene Barroy**, senior public finance expert, World Health Organization (WHO); **Piyush Bhutani**, consultant, ADB; **Robert Boothe**, principal planning and policy economist, ADB; **Kalipso Chalkidou**, director, Department of Health System Performance, Financing and Delivery, WHO; **Aekapol Chongvilaivan**, principal planning and policy economist, ADB; **Benjamin Coghlan**, consultant, ADB; **Santiago Cornejo**, executive manager, Regional Revolving Funds, PAHO; **Ramiro Guerrero**, principal specialist, Health Nutrition and Population Division, Inter-American Development Bank (IDB); **Javier Guzman**, chief, Health, Nutrition, and Population Division, IDB; **David Heymann**, professor, Infectious Disease Epidemiology, London School of Hygiene and Tropical Medicine (LSHTM); **Nansubuga Nagadya Isdahl**, consultant, ADB; **Philipp Kalpaxis**, principal procurement specialist, ADB; **Akiko Kitamura**, senior health specialist, ADB; **Frederik Kristensen**, managing director, Regionalized Vaccine Manufacturing Collaborative; **Jae Kyoun Kim**, health specialist, ADB; **Hoon Sang Lee**, chief strategy officer, RIGHT Foundation; **Cheryl Legaspi**, consultant, ADB; **Amanda McClelland**, senior vice-president of Prevent Epidemics at Resolve to Save Lives; **Matilde Neret**, principal operations specialist, Health, Nutrition and Population Division, IDB; **Blaire Ng**, health specialist, ADB; **Jesper Pedersen**, director, Procurement Division, ADB; **Rosanna Peeling**, professor emeritus, LSHTM; **Patricia Rhee**, assistant general counsel, ADB; **Sofia Shakil**, director, Human and Social Development, ADB; **Amandeep Singh**, senior social sector specialist, ADB; **Harkabir Singh Jandu**, director, Ending Violence Against Children, Children's Investment Fund Foundation; **Soumya Swaminathan**, chair, MS Swaminathan Research Foundation; **Anna Vassall**, Joep Lange Chair in Global Health Economics, University of Amsterdam; **Prashant Yadav**, senior fellow for Global Health, Council on Foreign Relations; and **Hui Yang**, head of supply operations, The Global Fund to Fight AIDS, Tuberculosis and Malaria.

ABBREVIATIONS

ADB	Asian Development Bank
ASEAN	Association of Southeast Asian Nations
CEPI	Coalition for Epidemic Preparedness Innovation
COVID-19	coronavirus disease
DMC	developing member country
HEPR	health emergency preparedness and response
IFI	international financial institution
IHR	International Health Regulations
LMIC	low- and middle-income country
MDB	multilateral development bank
ODA	official development assistance
PFM	public financial management
PPPR	pandemic prevention, preparedness, and response
R&D	research and development
UHC	universal health coverage
VTD	vaccine, therapeutic, and diagnostic
WHO	World Health Organization

CHAPTER 1

Introduction

More than 1,000 days since the World Health Organization (WHO) declared the coronavirus disease (COVID-19) pandemic over, many health systems remain ill-equipped to prevent or respond to another major outbreak. Countries continue to underspend on health because of fiscal constraints. Important developments in international cooperation, such as the Pandemic Fund and the WHO Pandemic Agreement, have been challenged by funding shortfalls and weak accountability mechanisms.[1] At the same time, the financing landscape for global health is undergoing significant change, demanding corresponding changes to health systems in low- and middle-income countries (LMICs)—available resources and new investments both need to be used more strategically.

In this context, multilateral development banks (MDBs) have an important role to play in strengthening health security within and across countries. As providers of long-term sovereign and nonsovereign financing, MDBs are uniquely positioned to link pandemic preparedness priorities with broader health system strengthening, climate resilience, and economic recovery objectives. In Asia and the Pacific, where disease spillover and cross-border risks are significant, there is a growing need to move beyond fragmented, short-term financing toward coordinated, investment-oriented approaches that can be sustained over time.

But where should financing be directed? What are the priority investments for governments, MDBs, and other funders? To answer these questions and to improve readiness for future pandemics, the Asian Development Bank (ADB) held a **Symposium on Multilateral Financing for Pandemic Preparedness and Response** in July 2025 as part of ADB's inaugural INclusive, Sustainable, Prosperous and REsilient (INSPIRE) Health Forum. The symposium brought together government leaders, multilateral banks, health experts, and industry partners to share insights on how to advance regional health security and pandemic preparedness through inclusive financing, stronger institutions, and sustained partnerships.

The symposium underscored two points: (i) the urgent need for sustainable financing for pandemic prevention, preparedness, and response (PPPR) or, more broadly, health emergency preparedness and response (HEPR); and (ii) the necessity of assuring timely and equitable access to vaccines, therapeutics, and diagnostics (VTDs). ADB has compiled papers from panelists at the symposium to propose an investment road map for financing priority actions for governments and international financial institutions (IFIs) across the different phases of the pandemic cycle. Rather than providing an exhaustive list of financing solutions, the manuscript focuses on how best to strengthen **strategic, financing, and governance** functions that allow for PPPR and the operational ecosystem for equitable access to VTDs.

1 The Pandemic Fund was launched in 2022 and is the first multilateral financing mechanism dedicated exclusively to strengthening critical PPPR capacities at the national, regional, and global levels, with a focus on LMICs. The WHO Pandemic Agreement, adopted in May 2025, sets out the principles, approaches, and tools for better international coordination across a range of areas to strengthen the global health architecture for PPPR.

Health systems that are prepared for and prevent pandemics (and health systems that are resilient to other threats, such as those related to climate change) are fundamentally linked to progress toward universal health coverage (UHC). Integrating HEPR with UHC strategies maximizes the impact of investments, strengthens routine and emergency care, and ensures that health security advances equity and sustainability for all.

This publication is divided into three parts.

Part I charts progress and recent developments in the PPPR ecosystem—noting gaps and shortcomings in the post-pandemic era; the enduring need to strengthen PPPR coordination, financing, and governance; and the role of governments, MDBs, and other institutions in ensuring sustainable financing for PPPR actions.

Part II takes a deeper dive into existing challenges in strategy, financing, and governance for PPPR and the value chain (ecosystem) for VTDs. Opportunities to close gaps and leverage lessons learned from COVID-19 and other outbreaks are explored.

Part III offers an ambitious road map to deliver potential PPPR investments.

The intended audience for this publication includes government officials, IFIs, international organizations, and other regional and global health stakeholders. It aims to translate important lessons into policy and investment actions, serving as a tool to increase sustainable financing flows for PPPR and to build more equitable, resilient health systems.

CHAPTER 2

Charting Progress

RECENT DEVELOPMENTS IN PANDEMIC PREPAREDNESS AND RESPONSE

Pandemic preparedness and response are global public goods that require collective investment in health systems.

The Lasting Legacy of COVID-19

The COVID-19 impact. COVID-19 has left a profound mark on the world. Between January 2020 and December 2023, WHO estimated that more than 14 million excess deaths occurred worldwide, with nearly half of them in Asia.[2] Other estimates suggest that the true number of global excess deaths since COVID-19 has exceeded 28 million.[3]

Disruptions in health services. During the peak of the crisis, health systems were overloaded, and vital services were paused. In more than 90% of countries surveyed by WHO, essential services including maternal and newborn care, childhood immunization, and noncommunicable disease management were disrupted.[4] Vaccination campaigns were paused, elective surgeries postponed, and diagnostic and preventive programs scaled back as facilities redirected staff and supplies to the emergency response. In South Asia, outpatient visits in some public hospitals dropped by more than 40% at the pandemic's height, and recovery has remained uneven across subregions.[5] Routine immunization coverage in Southeast Asia fell from 91% in 2019 to 83% in 2022, erasing nearly a decade of progress.[6]

Consequences in the global economy. The global economic fallout was equally severe. The International Monetary Fund estimates cumulative output losses of $12.5 trillion between 2020 and 2024, equivalent to almost 9% of pre-pandemic gross domestic product.[7] Economies of Asian developing countries collectively contracted by 0.7% in 2020, marking their first recession in 6 decades.[8] Tourism revenues plunged by over 70% in Pacific island economies (footnote 7). ADB estimates that 170 million jobs were lost across the region in 2020 alone, with women and informal-sector workers most affected.[9]

2 WHO. 2022. 14.9 Million Excess Deaths Associated with the COVID-19 Pandemic in 2020 and 2021. News release. 5 May.

3 H. Clark and E. Johnson Sirleaf. 2024. *No Time to Gamble: Leaders Must Unite to Prevent Pandemics.* The Independent Panel for Pandemic Preparedness and Response.

4 WHO. 2021. COVID-19 Continues to Disrupt Essential Health Services in 90% of Countries. News release. 23 April.

5 R. M. Manna et al. 2025. Impact of COVID-19 on In-Patient and Out-Patient Services in Bangladesh. *PLoS One*. 20 (2). e0315626.

6 WHO. 2023. Global Excess Deaths Associated with COVID-19 (Modelled Estimates). Data set (accessed 19 January 2026).

7 *CNBCTV18*. 2022. COVID-19: Total Losses Likely to Touch $13.8 Trillion by 2024, says IMF Chief Economist Gita Gopinath. 25 January.

8 ADB. 2020. *Asian Development Outlook 2020 Update: Wellness in Worrying Times.*

9 Y. Sawada and L. R. Sumulong. 2021. Macroeconomic Impact of COVID-19 in Developing Asia. *ADBI Working Paper Series*. No. 1251. Asian Development Bank Institute.

The resulting income collapse reversed years of poverty reduction gains, pushing tens of millions back below national poverty lines and increasing fiscal deficits and debt distress.[10] Countries are now servicing their debt at higher interest rates, with interest rates rising to an all-time high in 2023.[11] This comes at a time when official development assistance for health has declined, with the risk of crowding out critical investments in education, health, and infrastructure.

Socioeconomic effects. The socioeconomic consequences of the pandemic continue to persist. Labor force participation and productivity remain below pre-pandemic levels in many LMICs, while inflation-driven food and energy price shocks have exacerbated inequality. The Organisation for Economic Co-operation and Development (OECD) estimates that long COVID may be responsible for keeping 3 million people out of the workforce in OECD countries, with an annual cost of up to $1.04 trillion.[12] School closures, averaging 41 weeks in Asia, resulted in an estimated 0.8 learning-adjusted years of schooling lost per child.[13] The pandemic's intertwined health and socioeconomic effects underscored that the enduring scars from unprepared and weak health systems extend far beyond the health sector, with pervasive and stubborn disruptions to education, employment, and fiscal policy.

Asia and the Pacific at Risk

Shortfall in global pandemic financing. Global financing for PPPR continues to fall short of the need. Despite repeated calls for sustained investment, global health security financing continues to remain crisis-driven and inconsistent, spiking during emergencies but fading once the immediate threat has passed. Between 2016 and 2018, contributions to WHO's Contingency Fund for Emergencies fell by over 30%, reflecting the absence of predictable, multiyear funding streams.[14] A 2022 WHO–World Bank analysis estimated that only $4 billion–$5 billion was being invested annually in preparedness, compared with an estimated global requirement of $31 billion, including around $10 billion in external support for LMICs.[15] Further, the Pandemic Fund, launched in 2022, remains oversubscribed having received just $2.25 billion to date.[16] With official development assistance projected to decline by up to 17% in 2025, and potentially up to 40%–60% over the next 5 years,[17] plus an annual underfinancing for pandemic preparedness, LMICs will disproportionately bear the brunt of this shortfall in financing for health emergency preparedness.

Disparities in pandemic-related spending. Pandemic preparedness and response spending has significant disparities on a per capita basis.

10 International Monetary Fund. 2020. *Fiscal Monitor: Policies for the Recovery*; and International Monetary Fund. 2023. *IMF Annual Report 2023*.

11 World Bank. 2024. Developing Countries Paid Record $1.4 Trillion on Foreign Debt in 2023. Press release. 3 December.

12 A. Espinosa Gonzalez and E. Suzuki. 2024. The Impacts of Long COVID Across OECD Countries. *OECD Health Working Papers*. No. 167. OECD.

13 ADB. 2021. *Learning and Earning Losses from COVID-19 School Closures in Developing Asia*. Special Topic of the Asian Development Outlook 2021.

14 Global Preparedness Monitoring Board. 2019. *A World at Risk: GPMB 2019 Annual Report*.

15 WHO and World Bank. 2022. *Analysis of Pandemic Preparedness and Response (PPR) Architecture, Financing Needs, Gaps and Mechanisms*.

16 Independent Panel for Pandemic Preparedness and Response. 2025. *The Power to Lead for a Safer World*.

17 E. Barringer. 2025. A New Funding Paradigm for Global Health: Navigating the Sharp Decline in ODA. *Dahlberg*. May.

Among ADB members, spending levels and financing sources for PPPR vary.[18] Between 2019 and 2022, low-income countries spent between $1.2 and $2.9 per capita on PPPR, while lower-middle-income countries ranged from $1.8 to $7.7, and upper-middle-income countries from $7.7 to $20.8. High-income countries spent up to $140.5 per capita on PPPR in 2022—almost eight times more than upper-middle-income countries and 30 times more than lower-middle-income countries (Figure 1; country-specific data for 2022 are presented in Figure 2).

The sources of PPPR financing also largely vary. Some countries, such as Thailand and Fiji, rely predominantly on domestic resources to fund PPPR efforts (Figure 3). In contrast, others remain heavily dependent on external financing—for instance, the Lao People's Democratic Republic (80% of total PPPR spending is funded through external resources) and Myanmar (63%) in 2022. Countries such as the Republic of Korea, Thailand, and Viet Nam[19] demonstrated that prior investments in preparedness and prevention enabled a more effective and timely response (Box 1).

Figure 1: Per Capita Pandemic Prevention, Preparedness, and Response Spending by Income Level, 2019–2022

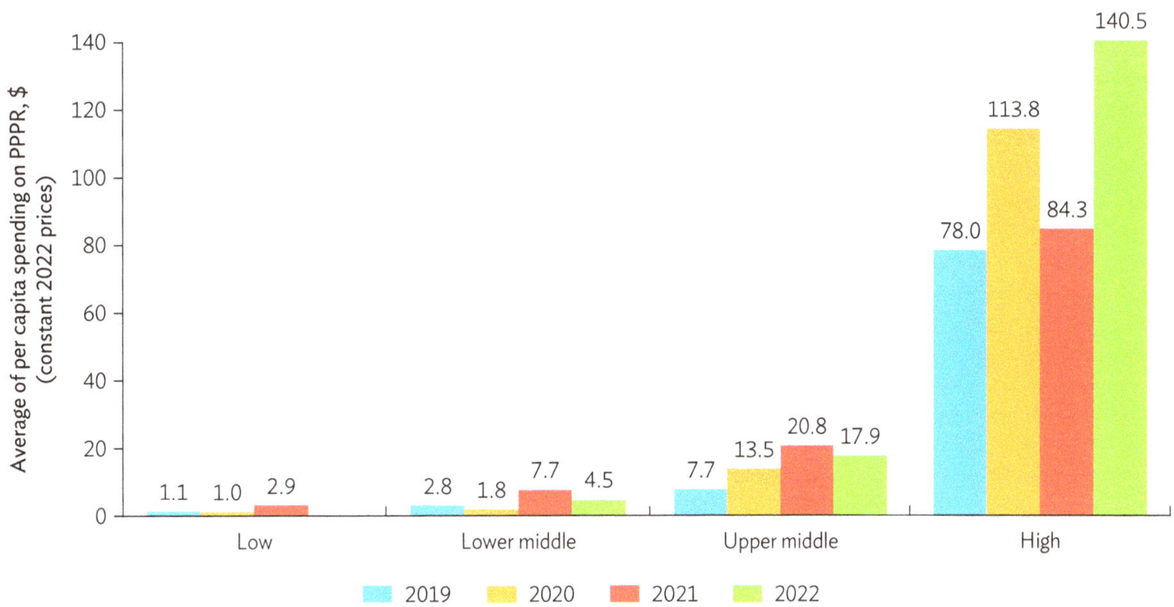

PPPR = pandemic prevention, preparedness, and response.

Source: World Health Organization. 2024. Global Health Expenditure Database.

18 The data analysis approach builds on the methodology used for the Group of 20 (G20) Joint Finance and Health Task Force report on PPPR financing released in 2025. Since many ADB members' budget tracking systems do not allow for direct identification of PPPR-specific spending, this report used data from the WHO Global Health Expenditure Database to estimate PPPR expenditures. This was done by applying the same allocation keys and shares as in the G20 report, but only for ADB members and only for years where data were available. Importantly, data are reported strictly based on availability in the WHO Global Health Expenditure Database—no extrapolations by income group have been conducted.

19 P. L. Osewe. 2021. *Pandemic Preparedness and Response Strategies: COVID-19 Lessons from the Republic of Korea, Thailand, and Viet Nam*. Asian Development Bank.

Figure 2: Per Capita Pandemic Prevention, Preparedness, and Response Spending in Selected Asian Development Bank Members by Income Level, 2019–2022

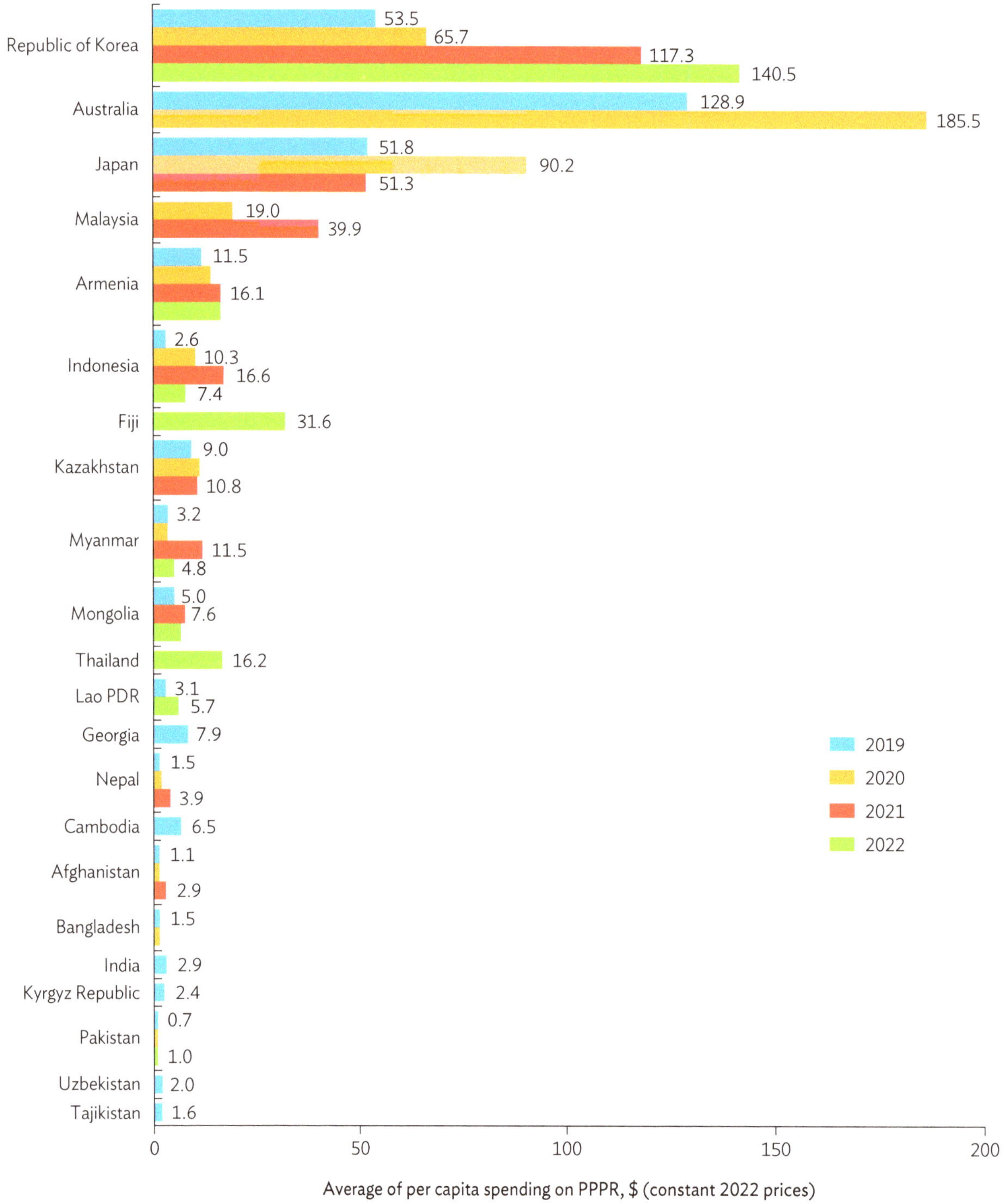

ADB = Asian Development Bank; Lao PDR = Lao People's Democratic Republic; PPPR = pandemic prevention, preparedness, and response.

Notes: (i) ADB placed its regular assistance to Afghanistan on hold effective 15 August 2021.
(ii) Effective 1 February 2021, ADB placed a temporary hold on sovereign project disbursements and new contracts in Myanmar.

Source: World Health Organization. 2024. Global Health Expenditure Database.

Figure 3: Sources of Pandemic Preparedness and Response Spending in Selected ADB Developing Member Countries

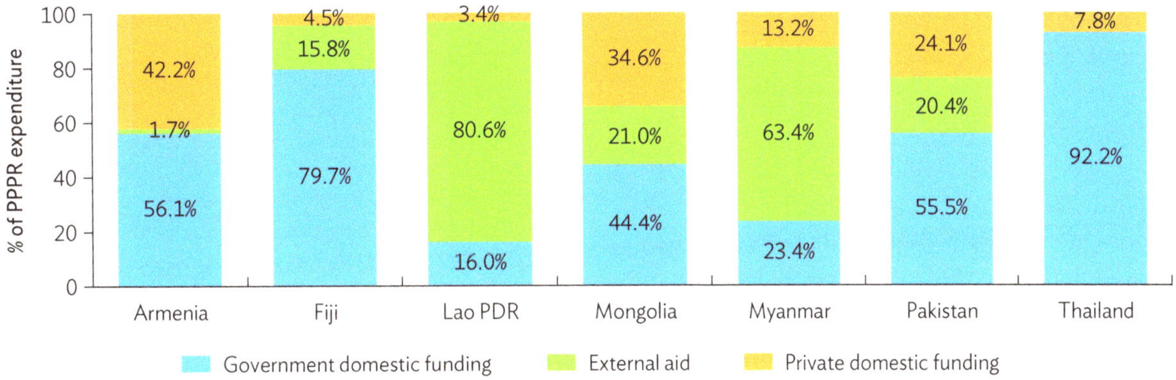

ADB = Asian Development Bank; Lao PDR = Lao People's Democratic Republic; PPPR = pandemic prevention, preparedness, and response.

Note: Effective 1 February 2021, ADB placed a temporary hold on sovereign project disbursements and new contracts in Myanmar.

Source: World Health Organization. 2024. Global Health Expenditure Database.

Box 1

Successful Health Response to COVID-19 Through Domestic Resources: The Case of Viet Nam

Viet Nam's successful response to the coronavirus disease (COVID-19) was underpinned by strong domestic resource mobilization and sustained investment in health system preparedness. Between 2019 and 2021, the government increased health spending significantly, allocating approximately $1.5 billion for pandemic response measures. These funds supported rapid scaling of testing, contact tracing, quarantine facilities, and public communication campaigns. Viet Nam's prior investments in surveillance systems, primary care infrastructure, and health workforce capacity—driven by lessons from past outbreaks—enabled swift and coordinated action. As a result, the country maintained one of the lowest COVID-19 case and mortality rates in the region during the early phases of the pandemic, demonstrating the critical role of domestic financing in building resilient health systems.

Source: P. L. Osewe. 2021. *Pandemic Preparedness and Response Strategies: COVID-19 Lessons from the Republic of Korea, Thailand, and Viet Nam.* Asian Development Bank.

Spending and financing gaps compounding weaknesses in global governance. The 2005 International Health Regulations (IHR), which are legally binding for all 196 WHO member states, require countries to build core capacities in surveillance, laboratory diagnostics, and risk communication. However, by 2019, fewer than 40% of countries had achieved even basic compliance with these requirements (footnote 13). Independent reviews of pandemic response during previous outbreaks pointed toward challenges such as delayed reporting, limited transparency, and insufficient authority to verify data. Moreover, pandemic preparedness was often siloed within health ministries, detached from the finance, trade, and defense sectors that determine national allocation of resources, despite the evidence that even modest investments in preparedness can yield much larger returns (Box 2). Even as the global health security agenda and global frameworks have expanded and major milestones have been achieved—such as the adoption of the Pandemic Agreement in May 2025, amendments to the IHR in September of 2025, a new Coordinating

Financial Mechanism to be established under the IHR and Pandemic Agreement (footnote 15), and the release of the Group of 20 (G20) World Bank–WHO Operational Playbook for Pandemic Response Financing[20]—compliance, accountability, and sustained leadership remain fragmented and at risk.[21]

Underinvestment and institutional fragmentation making Asia and the Pacific vulnerable. Most LMICs in the region lack the fiscal space to maintain surveillance, workforce, and emergency-response functions between crises, relying on disjointed donor projects rather than stable domestic allocations. Without preparedness embedded in national budgets and multilateral frameworks, countries in Asia and the Pacific have remained locked in a cycle of reactive spending, delayed mobilization, and chronic vulnerability. While high-income economies in the region built advanced surveillance networks, many LMICs struggled to maintain routine laboratory and emergency-response operations. Regional mechanisms such as the Association of Southeast Asian Nations (ASEAN) Disease Outbreak Response System of Systems, COVID-19 ASEAN Response Fund, and the World Health Organization South-East Asia Regional Health Emergency Fund reflect progress, yet lack sustainable financing and interoperability with global frameworks. As a result, the region entered 2020 with strong technical expertise but limited fiscal flexibility, coordination capacity, and supply-chain resilience.

Equitable access to vaccine, therapeutic, and diagnostics (VTDs)—a strategic necessity. During the COVID-19 pandemic, countries across the world, including in Asia and the Pacific, were effectively blocked from procurement of vaccines. This was largely due to individual agreements between high-income countries and manufacturers and a lack of transparency, which resulted in unequal distribution. Other factors contributing to vaccine inequity included gaps in production capacity, regulatory agility, and data governance. Accelerated vaccine development demonstrated the enormous potential of global collaboration; however, the absence of harmonized regulatory standards and technology-transfer mechanisms perpetuated delays across LMICs. Regionalized and subregionalized approaches to rapidly scale manufacturing of VTDs and achieve self-reliance for VTDs are gaining prominence in Asia and the Pacific.

Box 2

The Economic Case for Preparedness

Multiple simulated and empirical studies strengthen the case that preparedness delivers high returns. Annual global preparedness needs are estimated between $24.8 billion and $43 billion, with every dollar invested in pandemic preparedness for a coronavirus disease (COVID-19)-like pandemic scenario yielding $1,703 in health gains and $1,102 in economic gains, while averting 49 to 124 deaths per 100,000 population. In the context of emerging diseases, cross-sector investments in prevention, which is underfinanced even relative to preparedness or response, can pay off many times—annual prevention cost have been estimated at under 1% of the costs to respond to COVID-19 in 2020.

Sources:

Center for Global Development. 2021. *What is the Return on Investment of Pandemic Preparedness?* CDG Talks Event. Washington, DC. 4 October.

L. Clarke et al. 2022. The Costs of Improving Health Emergency Preparedness: A Systematic Review and Analysis of Multi-Country Studies. *eClinicalMedicine*. 44. 101269.

World Bank. 2022. *Putting Pandemics Behind Us: Investing in One Health to Reduce Risks of Emerging Infectious Diseases.*

World Health Organization and World Bank. 2022. *Analysis of Pandemic Preparedness and Response (PPR) Architecture, Financing Needs, Gaps and Mechanisms.*

[20] G20 Brasil 2024. Finance Track: Joint Task Force on Finance and Health.

[21] H. Barroy, K. Chalkidou, and S. Gupta. 2025. Financing for Future Pandemics: Three Strategic Shifts We Need Now. Blog post. Center for Global Development. 24 September.

Changing Context

Proactive preparedness and moving beyond ad hoc responses. The pandemic revealed that preparedness cannot rely on episodic emergency measures or donor-driven projects. COVID-19 showcased how countries that had invested consistently in prevention and epidemiology training—such as Singapore's integrated risk-communication systems or Viet Nam's field epidemiology programs—managed to contain early outbreak waves effectively. Going forward, preparedness must be treated as a standing public good, funded through multiyear domestic allocations and embedded within fiscal frameworks rather than as ad hoc responses. Regular stress testing of national health-security capacities through simulation exercises, linked to expenditure reviews and debt-sustainability analyses, can also help governments balance preventive spending with macro-fiscal discipline.

Sustainable financing of health emergencies. There is a requirement for a structural transformation in how countries—and organizations—prepare for, govern, and finance health emergencies. The COVID-19 crisis has reinforced the notion that prevention and preparedness are whole-of-government, whole-of-society responsibilities, not splintered sector functions. Those countries that had lower mortality during the COVID-19 pandemic had, for example, (i) health care systems that could accommodate both those requiring routine care and the extra caseload of patients with severe acute respiratory syndrome coronavirus 2 (SARS-CoV-2) infections and complications; (ii) strong public health systems with surveillance and response capacities, such as outbreak investigation and contact tracing; and (iii) effective health promotion arms resulting in populations with fewer co-morbidities, lower susceptibility to serious disease, and trust in vaccines. This, therefore, calls for urgent realignment of strategic, financing, and governance frameworks to meet evolving demands and deliver effective and agile pandemic solutions. Crucially, but not exclusively, this includes creating sustainable pathways to equitable production, procurement, and distribution of VTDs.

Acknowledging the broader importance of health systems. The aftermath of COVID-19 has catalyzed a fundamental shift in how governments, IFIs, and development partners conceive of health systems. The pandemic revealed that health is not a self-contained social sector but a critical pillar of economic stability, fiscal sustainability, and resilience-building across sectors. This realization is reshaping investment logic across the multilateral system, adding new impetus to the transition from vertical, disease-specific interventions to integrated, systems-based financing that link health security to broader development goals, including interconnected challenges such as social protection, climate resilience, and environmental sustainability.

The interdependence of preparedness, UHC, and economic resilience—an emerging paradigm. Health systems must therefore be designed not only to deliver care but to absorb and adapt to disruptions from pandemics, climate events, economic crises, and other shocks. WHO's 2024 Health Systems Resilience Framework (Box 3) articulates this as the capacity to "absorb, adapt, and transform."[22] Countries such as Thailand and the Republic of Korea demonstrated that strong primary-care networks, digital surveillance platforms, and prepositioned emergency-operations centers enable rapid containment without compromising essential services and with shorter society-wide lockdowns compared to most countries.

[22] WHO. 2022. *Health Systems Resilience Toolkit: A WHO Global Public Health Good to Support Building and Strengthening of Sustainable Health Systems Resilience in Countries with Various Contexts.*

Box 3

World Health Organization's Health Emergency Preparedness, Response, and Resilience Framework

The World Health Organization's Health Emergency Preparedness, Response, and Resilience framework, introduced in 2023, has identified five core systems for health emergency prevention, preparedness, response, and resilience. The five Cs focus on an ecosystem approach that revolve around the intersection of health security, primary health care and health promotion, and their interface with other sectors:

- **C**ollaborative surveillance,
- **C**ommunity protection,
- safe and scalable **C**are,
- access to **C**ountermeasures, and
- emergency **C**oordination.

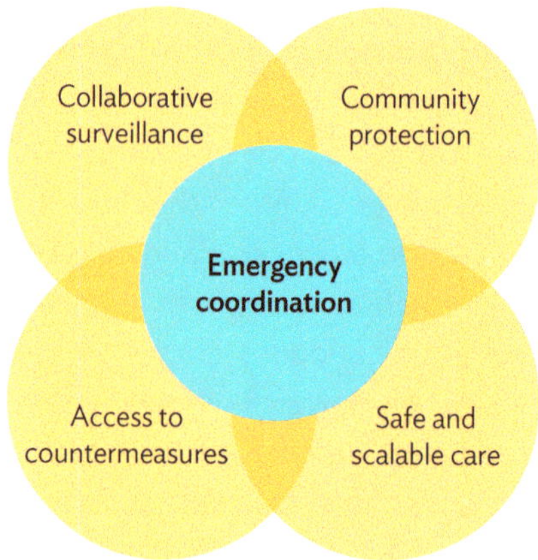

Source: World Health Organization. 2022. Strengthening the Global Architecture for Health Emergency Preparedness, Response and Resilience. Report by the Director-General. Seventy-Fifth World Health Assembly. Provisional Agenda Item 16.

Aligning of IFIs' operational models with the resilience agenda. The World Bank's HEPR Program[23] and ADB's recent investments in Mongolia, Sri Lanka, and Pacific island countries embed preparedness indicators directly into sovereign lending frameworks. These programs finance laboratory networks, digital-health architecture, climate-resilient hospital design, and workforce surge capacity under government budget systems rather than donor silos.
By treating preparedness as part of fiscal planning and public-investment management, IFIs help countries shift from reactive aid dependence to long-term system ownership, while at the same time strengthening routine functions such as public health surveillance and disease prevention.

Integrating climate and health financing. The integration of financing of preventive measures for climate change and health marks another inflection point. The intensifying climate crisis is amplifying vector-borne and zoonotic diseases, extreme-weather injuries, and nutrition-related morbidity. The World Bank estimates that without adaptive investment, climate-related health shocks could cause 15 million excess deaths and $20.8 trillion in economic losses in LMICs over the next quarter-century.[24] In response, IFIs are embedding health resilience into climate-finance pipelines. The 2023 G20 Delhi Declaration formally recognized climate and health as a shared global priority,[25] and IFIs have begun integrating "green health" metrics into project appraisal frameworks.

23 World Bank. Health Emergency Preparedness and Response Umbrella Program.

24 World Bank. 2024. *The Cost of Inaction: Quantifying the Impact of Climate Change on Health in Low- and Middle-Income Countries.*

25 G20 Member Nations. 2023. *G20 New Delhi Leaders' Declaration.* New Delhi. 9–10 September.

This includes indicators for renewable energy systems for hospitals, decarbonized supply chains, and flood-resilient infrastructure, among others. This approach reframes health spending as a dual-purpose investment that yields both adaptation and emission-reduction co-benefits. Relatedly, ADB has published a new comprehensive approach to protecting communities and their environment for projects it finances that encompasses environmental, health, social, cultural and other safeguards.[26]

Financial innovation underpinning this transformation. IFIs are piloting blended-finance models that combine concessional funds, guarantees, and private capital to expand fiscal space for health security. Instruments such as debt-for-health swaps, impact-linked financing, and contingent credit lines allow countries to access liquidity rapidly when outbreaks occur while preserving solvency. ADB's Contingent Disaster Financing Program releases funds automatically upon verified disaster thresholds, enabling countries to secure "always-on" preparedness financing without adding unsustainable debt. ADB's guarantee-based Innovative Finance Facility for Climate offers a relevant model for health: the guarantee-based structure multiplies concessional resources by up to five times, freeing balance-sheet space for crisis response.[27] Similar contingent finance mechanisms could be applied to health, establishing preapproved pandemic credit lines, countercyclical reserves, and parametric insurance triggers that release funds promptly upon verified disease outbreak thresholds.

The Evolving Role of Multilateral Development Banks

Leveraging comparative advantage. MDBs and IFIs occupy a unique position in the global pandemic preparedness and response architecture. Their financial scale, policy leverage, and country partnerships make them critical for operationalizing preparedness as a development priority. MDBs can convert technical regulations and international agreements into finance, fiscal integration, and implementation pathways. COVID-19 illustrated this complementarity where MDBs deployed over $200 billion in emergency health and social protection financing between 2020 and 2022, cushioning fiscal shocks and supporting vaccine access in over 150 countries (Figure 4 summarizes ADB's response to the COVID-19 pandemic).[28]

Correcting the asymmetry in investments in preparedness. Less vulnerable high-income economies invest substantially more in preparedness than low-income economies (Figure 1).[29] MDBs can reduce this inequity by pooling financing and providing predictable disbursement mechanisms. Their engagement also strengthens country ownership by embedding preparedness within fiscal frameworks rather than donor projects, transforming short-term crisis relief into long-term resilience.

Strategic partners for health sector resilience. MDBs and other IFIs are critical partners in building resilient health systems. A key gap in ADB's response during COVID-19 was its inability to implement advance purchase agreements with vaccine manufacturers ("at-risk procurement") for products that did not have the necessary regulatory approvals.

26 ADB. 2024. *Environmental and Social Framework.*

27 ADB. 2025. *IF-CAP: Innovative Finance Facility for Climate in Asia and the Pacific.*

28 N. Lee and R. Aboneaaj. 2021. MDB COVID-19 Crisis Response: Where Did the Money Go? *CGD Note.* Center for Global Development. November.

29 C. Penn et al. 2025. Smart Spending to Combat Global Health Threats: Tracking Expenditure on Prevention, Preparedness, and Response, and Other Global Public Goods for Health. *OECD Health Working Papers*. No. 175. OECD.

Figure 4: From Crisis to Recovery—ADB's Comprehensive Response to the COVID-19 Pandemic, 2020–2023

During the COVID-19 pandemic, ADB responded swiftly, demonstrating agility in supporting its DMCs. Its comprehensive response to the pandemic provided a $20 billion support package and introduced special policy variations such as the CPRO under the Countercyclical Support Facility, which provided crucial budget support to 27 DMCs. ADB's response also included APVAX, which helped DMCs procure and distribute COVID-19 vaccines, as well as enhance their systems for vaccine delivery and preparedness. Both the CPRO and APVAX helped strengthen DMCs' collective response to the pandemic and delivered cross-border as well as national benefits. ADB continues to support DMCs in their long-term solutions for pandemic preparedness and plans toward recovery.

During 2020–2023, total financing reached $68.9 billion, including $41.2 billion in ADB commitments and $27.7 billion in cofinancing, with collaborations reaching more than 100 organizations. Based on the ADB Client Perceptions Survey 2022, about 92% of ADB's primary clients rated ADB's overall performance positively in minimizing the adverse effects of COVID-19, and 95% believed that the impact made in their country with ADB support to address COVID-19 was "excellent," "good," or "satisfactory."

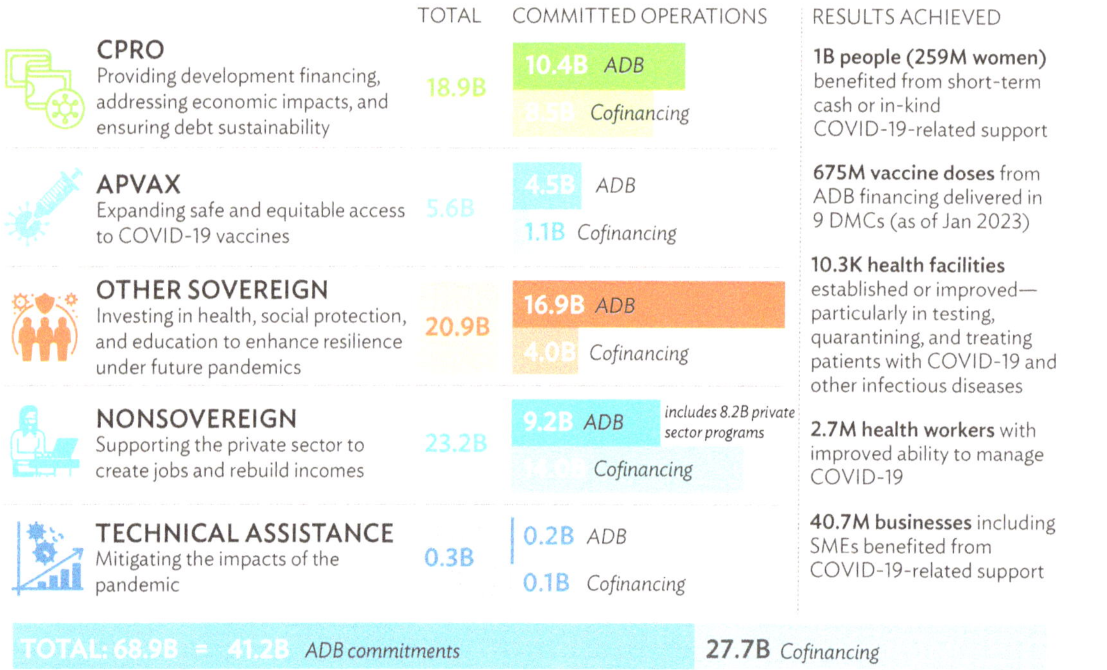

ADB = Asian Development Bank, APVAX = Asia Pacific Vaccine Access Facility, B = billion, COVID-19 = coronavirus disease, CPRO = COVID-19 Pandemic Response Option, DMC = developing member country, K = thousand, M = million, SMEs = small and medium-sized enterprises.

Sources: ADB. 2024. *Strategy 2030 Midterm Review: An Evolution Approach for the Asian Development Bank*; ADB. 2020. *ADB's Comprehensive Response to the COVID-19 Pandemic*; ADB. 2020. *ADB's Support to Enhance COVID-19 Vaccine Access*; ADB. ADB Client Perceptions Survey 2022. Unpublished; and various ADB reports.

It also had limited capacity to tackle fundamental weaknesses in developing member countries (DMCs) that impacted on timely COVID-19 responses (e.g., the maturity level of national regulators in the region), underscoring the idea that pandemic preparedness and response require more than just a financing role; it demands several interlinked activities to happen synchronously, many of which have long lead times. MDBs must move beyond financing, building more robust partnerships with technical actors and establishing cross-sector country platforms that convene ministries of finance, health, and environment, and the private sector to jointly plan and monitor investments (ADB in Action 1).

ADB in Action 1

A Timely and Strategic Response to COVID-19—Building on Lessons Learned

1. The **Regional Support to Address the Outbreak of Coronavirus Disease (COVID-19) and Potential Outbreaks of Other Communicable Diseases** technical assistance project was approved in February 2020 and was designed to rapidly address the demands of developing member countries (DMCs) for immediate emergency health assistance, including the procurement of personal protective equipment, medical equipment, and supplies. As the COVID-19 pandemic continued, assistance was expanded to provide financing and technical support to DMCs for health systems strengthening including assessments, vaccine deployments, and broader pandemic preparedness and response actions.

2. The **Asia Diagnostics, Vaccines, and Therapeutics Network to Counter Epidemics (ADVaNCE)** was launched in 2024 to bring together ministries of health, national regulatory authorities, manufacturers, academic institutions, and international organizations to build a coordinated regional approach to the development, regulation, and delivery of medical countermeasures. ADVaNCE operates through five strategic pillars that reflect the interconnected functions needed for resilient health systems capable of preparing and responding to future disease outbreaks and pandemics:
   - **Rapid response to pandemics:** Strengthening the region's collective readiness to produce, manufacture, and distribute essential vaccines, diagnostics, and therapeutics during emergencies.
   - **Regulatory capacity building:** Enhancing institutional capability, technical expertise, and governance to improve the quality and efficiency of regulatory oversight.
   - **Regulatory harmonization and convergence:** Aligning regulatory processes and standards across countries to facilitate faster, more predictable market access for quality-assured products.
   - **Collaborative procurement of medical countermeasures:** Developing mechanisms for joint purchasing to secure reliable, affordable, and timely supply during both routine and emergency situations.
   - **Local manufacturing:** Supporting technology transfer, quality management systems, and investments that enable sustainable regional production capacity.

3. The **Strengthening Regulatory Ecosystem and Manufacturing for Vaccines, Therapeutics, and Diagnostics in Asia and the Pacific (REVITALIZE)** project stimulates policy dialogue and financing to help countries operationalize ADVaNCE priorities. It is creating an enabling environment for resilient supply chains, strengthened regulatory systems, and regional manufacturing networks.

4. The **Ending Complex and Challenging Infectious and Tropical Diseases (ExCITD)** project aims to accelerate malaria elimination, reduce the tuberculosis (TB) burden, and improve dengue control. Asia and the Pacific have had mixed progress on tackling malaria; the region is home to two-thirds of global TB cases and 12 of the world's 30 high-burden countries; and sharp surges in dengue are testing health systems throughout the tropics. ExCITD will invest in early warning systems, digital surveillance, and climate-informed risk modeling, building the core capacities needed to detect and respond to emerging threats. The initiative will also pilot innovative interventions, such as Wolbachia replacement for dengue suppression and gender-responsive TB screening tools, accelerating regulatory adoption of new technologies, and fostering rapid scale-up through public–private partnerships. Sustainable financing—including concessional and blended mechanisms—is core to the project to ensure that outbreak preparedness and response investments are embedded in national budgets and long-term strategies.

Source: Asian Deve k. 2025. Symposium on Multilateral Financing for Pandemic Preparedness and Response. 1st INSPIRE Health Forum. ADB Headquarters, Manila. 11 July.

CHAPTER 3

Opportunities to Scale Up Pandemic Investment and Financing Priorities

A truly coherent approach to pandemic preparedness and response requires coordinated shifts across strategic, financing, governance, and security functions—at global, regional, and national levels.

Strengthening Pandemic Preparedness and Response Across Strategic, Financing, and Governance Functions

Pandemics emerge and persist because of inequities

STRATEGIC GAPS AND OPPORTUNITIES

- **Embedding pandemic preparedness and response into the global, national, and regional security architecture**

Pandemics—health shocks as well as global, regional, and national security threats. Pandemics can destabilize economies, strain political systems, and trigger cascading risks that spread across borders. Financing for preparedness must therefore be understood as part of the world's security architecture. The rationale is straightforward: just as countries invest in defense to guard against military threats, they must invest in resilient health systems that are able to support routine health needs and rapidly detect or prevent pandemics. At the same time, they must precommit resources to promptly respond and avoid preventable human and economic costs. This may require treating pandemic preparedness financing as a separate line of security spending, not simply as an extension of health budgets. Infrastructure, human resources, and training, such as in epidemiology, as well as protective equipment and other critical supplies, and countermeasures like vaccines, therapeutics, and diagnostics (VTDs) must all be included.

Ideally, financing for VTDs should encompass "at-risk" investments made before products are fully proven, so that supplies are accessible as soon as possible. Access to supplies and countermeasures during a pandemic must not depend on a country's fiscal space but on collective safeguards that reach all populations; thus, multicountry and regional approaches are increasingly being sought. For example, building scalable vaccine manufacturing capacity in hubs like Singapore or the Republic of Korea may not top local development agendas, but could be critical for national and regional security, given that smaller countries are less likely to impose and sustain export bans. By embedding pandemic preparedness and response financing in both national and regional security considerations, Asia and the Pacific can ensure that the next outbreak is met with an equitable response that shortens or even avoids crises.

- **Integrating pandemic preparedness and response into health system resilience**

Health system resilience—the foundation of preparedness. During COVID-19, 90% of countries reported disruptions to essential care (footnote 2). This interruption revealed that surge capacity must be built on strong primary care and public health systems.

Resilience requires sustained investment in six "core capacities" identified by WHO and the Joint External Evaluation: emergency coordination, surveillance, laboratory systems, workforce, logistics, and risk communication. Resilience also requires a workforce well trained in epidemiology and public health; clinical patient management that evolves in a pandemic as new evidence emerges; infection prevention and control; and incident management. For Asia and the Pacific, priorities include integrating preparedness metrics into universal health coverage (UHC) plans, financing climate-resilient and epidemic-ready health infrastructure, and establishing protected budgets for emergency logistics and workforce surge.

Prioritizing pandemic preparedness and response and universal health coverage investment co-benefits

Co-benefits from PPPR investments. Investments in pandemic prevention, preparedness, and response (PPPR) yield significant co-benefits and efficiencies. Ample evidence shows that many PPPR interventions—such as integrated surveillance systems, laboratory networks, and emergency logistics, underpinned by a workforce trained in applied epidemiology (Box 4)—also strengthen routine health services and improve responses to endemic diseases. For example, investments in collaborative surveillance can enhance detection of both pandemic-prone and endemic pathogens, avoiding the inefficiencies of parallel systems. Similarly, strengthening national public health institutes and data systems supports both emergency preparedness and day-to-day health service delivery (Figure 5). To ensure that PPPR investments are cost-effective and do not crowd out other health priorities, countries should integrate them into existing priority-setting and health technology assessment processes. This includes applying structured tools—such as multipayer economic evaluations—to compare the long-term benefits of PPPR interventions with more immediate health needs. Such tools help governments make trade-offs and allocate resources where they can achieve the greatest impact. Embedding emergency readiness within routine service delivery—rather than creating stand-alone vertical programs—can reduce duplication and build resilience across the system. For example, integrating emergency response protocols into primary care facilities ensures continuity of care during crises while enabling rapid scale-up when needed. Similarly, community engagement and trust-building are critical to both routine health delivery and emergency response, reinforcing the social foundations of resilience.

Box 4

Supporting Strategic Workforce Development for Pandemic Preparedness and Response

Strong primary health care systems facilitate early detection and rapid respond to public health crises, potentially averting large-scale outbreaks through localized action. The clinical suspicion of frontline health workers—the moment they recognize something unusual—is often our earliest warning of an outbreak. They can relay community concerns upward and tailor disease detection and control strategies to local realities. This vertical integration ensures that public health policy is grounded in the working realities of its frontline staff and the lived experience of the communities it serves. Although traditional definitions of primary health care include components that would help detect and respond to epidemics, this has often been overlooked. Investing in aspects of epidemic-ready primary health care (e.g., infection control, disease reporting, continuity of operations in an emergency) can be viewed as a safeguard not a cost—an insurance policy against the societal disruption that pandemics can unleash. For primary health care to effectively serve this crucial role, **health workers must be safe, equipped, and supported**.

Source: Resolve to Save Lives. Epidemic-Ready Primary Health Care.

Figure 5: Pandemic Prevention, Preparedness, and Response and Health System Investment Co-Benefits

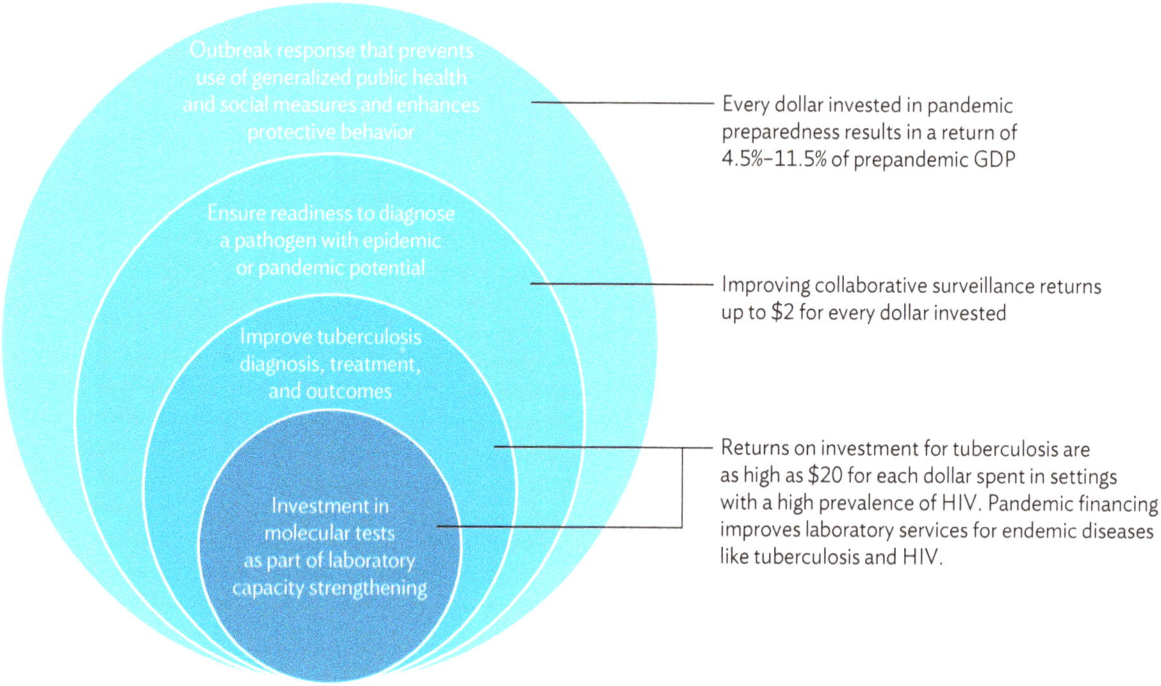

GDP = gross domestic product.

Source: Adapted from the G20 Joint Finance and Health Task Force report on pandemic prevention, preparedness, and response financing.

Several ADB-supported initiatives, such as the Greater Mekong Subregion Health Security Project and regional disease surveillance networks, demonstrate how preparedness investments can yield crosscutting benefits for routine service delivery, health workforce development, and digital health infrastructure. ADB's Ending Complex and Challenging Infectious and Tropical Diseases (ExCITD) initiative is a practical example of how disease-focused efforts can be integrated with system-wide PPPR efforts, climate adaptation strategies, and routine health care systems (ADB in Action 1). Scaling such models across the region, while embedding them in national planning and budgeting processes, can help ensure that PPPR financing delivers both immediate value and long-term resilience.

For ADB's lower-income members, many of which face constrained fiscal space and competing budget priorities, maximizing the efficiency and co-benefits of PPPR investments is particularly critical. The region's diversity—ranging from small island states to large middle-income economies—requires context-specific approaches that integrate PPPR into broader health system and UHC strategies.

Advancing surveillance

Cost-effective pandemic defenses—early detection and transparent information sharing. Early detection and transparent information sharing remain the most cost-effective form of pandemic defense.

Despite progress, gaps in surveillance, genomic sequencing, and data exchange persist. By 2023, fewer than one-third of low-income countries had capacity to link genomic data with clinical and epidemiologic surveillance in real time.[30] The Global Influenza Surveillance and Response System, the genomic surveillance system of the Global Polio Eradication Initiative, WHO's Epidemic Intelligence Hub (Berlin), the Food and Agriculture Organization's Global Early Warning System for Major Animal Diseases, and the Pathogen Access and Benefit-Sharing System envisioned under the Pandemic Agreement represent milestones toward an integrated global network. For Asia and the Pacific, advancing collaborative surveillance systems means establishing interoperable regional platforms that integrate human, animal, and environmental health ("One Health") data into risk assessment (Box 5).[31] ASEAN's Health Cluster 2, ADB's One Health Framework (2023–2027), and the ASEAN Regional Public Health Laboratory Network are critical building blocks. Investments should prioritize the following: (i) real-time digital surveillance infrastructure, including data-sharing platforms; (ii) secure data standards with cross-border interoperability; and (iii) genomic and epidemiologic workforce training.

▸ Investing in diagnostics—a critical but undervalued tool

Diagnostics—essential for new and old pathogens. Without diagnostics, health systems are blind to new (and old) pathogens. Diagnostics are the first tool to understand the cause of an illness, its distribution in a population and, increasingly, disease control options including treatments, vaccines, and public health interventions. Connected diagnostic and laboratory infrastructure form the backbone of a health care system: sounding alarms of unusual disease patterns, sending early outbreak alerts, and monitoring the effectiveness of the response. In countries with robust health data systems and connectivity, they can provide real-time intelligence (e.g., monitoring supply chains). However, diagnostics are often undervalued and viewed as a cost to the health system; the consequence is chronic underinvestment. Appropriate diagnostic tests—from regional and national reference labs down to the community level—are indispensable for health security and help foster public trust, particularly as diagnostics move from health practitioner-administered and fixed facilities into mobile and home settings with diagnostics administered by lay people.

Box 5

A Risk-Based Approach

Financing for preparedness and response is too often bundled into broad development or health budgets without earmarking for surveillance, diluting its purpose. A **risk-based perspective** is needed: investing heaviest in health systems where new pathogens are most likely to emerge and where early containment can deliver great global benefit, while understanding that the emergence of a pandemic organism is a random event, making it important for all countries to sustain basic investments in core areas such as surveillance, infection prevention and control, and biosecurity. Directing even modest investments strategically can improve the chances that outbreaks can be stopped from escalating into global crises—averting trillions in losses and protecting lives and livelihoods.

Source: The Pandemic Fund. 2026. *Risk-Need Metric and Methodology: A Methodology for Identifying High Risk and High Need Countries Where Outbreaks Could Escalate into Pandemics.*

30 A. S. Gonzalez-Reiche. 2023. SARS-CoV-2 in Low-Income Countries: The Need for Sustained Genomic Surveillance. *The Lancet Global Health*. 11 (6). e815–e816.

31 WHO. 2023. *Defining Collaborative Surveillance: A Core Concept for Strengthening the Global Architecture for Health Emergency Preparedness, Response, and Resilience (HEPR).*

Like vaccines, the regulation of diagnostics was a bottleneck during the COVID-19 pandemic. Hundreds of brands of COVID-19 tests were developed and commercialized and yet the availability of diagnostics in many countries was delayed because of regulatory and policy barriers. Promoting regulatory reliance, convergence and harmonization, joint health technology assessments, and joint regulatory–policy assessments—in which regulators and policymakers hold joint review with subject matter experts to make critical decisions on test accuracy and the quality of manufacturing—can accelerate access to diagnostics for pandemic and routine use.

Regional mechanisms offer efficient ways to simplify and streamline these processes, public–private partnerships that stitch together demand and supply for diagnostics could stabilize manufacturing capacity, and a regionalized approach to diagnostic manufacturing could follow that being encouraged for pandemic vaccines (Box 6 and Box 13). One of the challenges in enlisting private sector interest in diagnostics for diseases of epidemic potential is the inconsistent demand for these products—low in inter-epidemic periods and huge during epidemics. One solution is to ensure a stable market by countries jointly developing a regional surveillance framework for high-priority diseases with defined annual test volumes (akin to an advanced bulk purchase commitment), combined with projections for future pandemics. This approach facilitates scale-up of manufacturing when needed, given tests are in regular production. It also aligns diagnostic supplies with the incremental strengthening of national and regional surveillance systems required under the International Health Regulations (IHR). Behind these processes lie a workforce versed in regulatory science and clinical trials—skills missing in most countries.

Box 6

Protecting the Most Vulnerable Countries and Scaling Regional Solutions

Despite overall investments in coronavirus disease (COVID-19) responses in the trillions of dollars and unprecedented scientific cooperation, the world delivered an inequitable response: low-income countries reached an average full vaccination coverage of 28% by November 2023, a year and a half after high-income countries had achieved 40% coverage. This inequity was due in large part to wealthy countries securing advance purchase agreements with manufacturers with up-front payments, permitting industry to rapidly scale up existing vaccine development and licensing. While the Pandemic Agreement sets the path to greater vaccine equity, challenges remain. For instance, there are concerns about data sharing and the benefits that come from sharing data, and the agreement lacks concrete funding commitments and enforcement mechanisms. Notably, the Pandemic Agreement encourages countries to align existing global and regional financing entities, such as the Pandemic Fund, Gavi, and the Global Fund, to reduce duplication and maximize impact.

More investments are needed in universal health coverage, primary health care, operationalizing One Health, and mitigating and preventing the socioeconomic inequalities that are drivers of pandemics. Social protection schemes (e.g., social safety nets, unemployment protection, and food security) are essential to minimize the wide-ranging social and economic damage of pandemics and ensuring equitable recovery. Multilateral development banks play an important role in catalyzing immediate and long-term pandemic prevention, preparedness, and response solutions that are designed to work in concert with broader social investments at the country-level. Similarly, multilateral development banks can finance regional integration and cooperation initiatives that improve common goods for pandemic prevention, preparedness, and response such as regulatory harmonization, coordinated national health security plans and policies, collaborative procurement mechanisms for medical countermeasures and equitable distribution of vaccines, therapeutics, and diagnostics.

Source: Soumya Swaminathan. 2025. Symposium on Multilateral Financing for Pandemic Preparedness. INSPIRE Health Forum. Manila.

Pandemics begin and end in communities

FINANCING GAPS AND OPPORTUNITIES

▸ Anchoring pandemic prevention, preparedness, and response in sustainable public financing

Domestic revenue—the key to sustainable PPPR financing. Sustainable financing for PPPR requires increased domestic revenue mobilization. Across ADB's DMCs, the COVID-19 pandemic catalyzed a temporary surge in domestic health spending, with many governments mobilizing public resources through budget reprioritization and emergency allocations. However, this momentum has proven difficult to sustain. By 2022, domestic public spending on health in several low-income and lower-middle-income countries had declined to below the average total government expenditure of 7% for these income groups (Figure 6). This decline in budget prioritization reflects both fiscal tightening and the reemergence of competing budgetary pressures. At the same time, debt-servicing obligations have increasingly constrained fiscal space, particularly where external debt burdens have outpaced health sector allocations.

Figure 6: Budget Prioritization for Health in ADB's Developing Member Countries, 2022

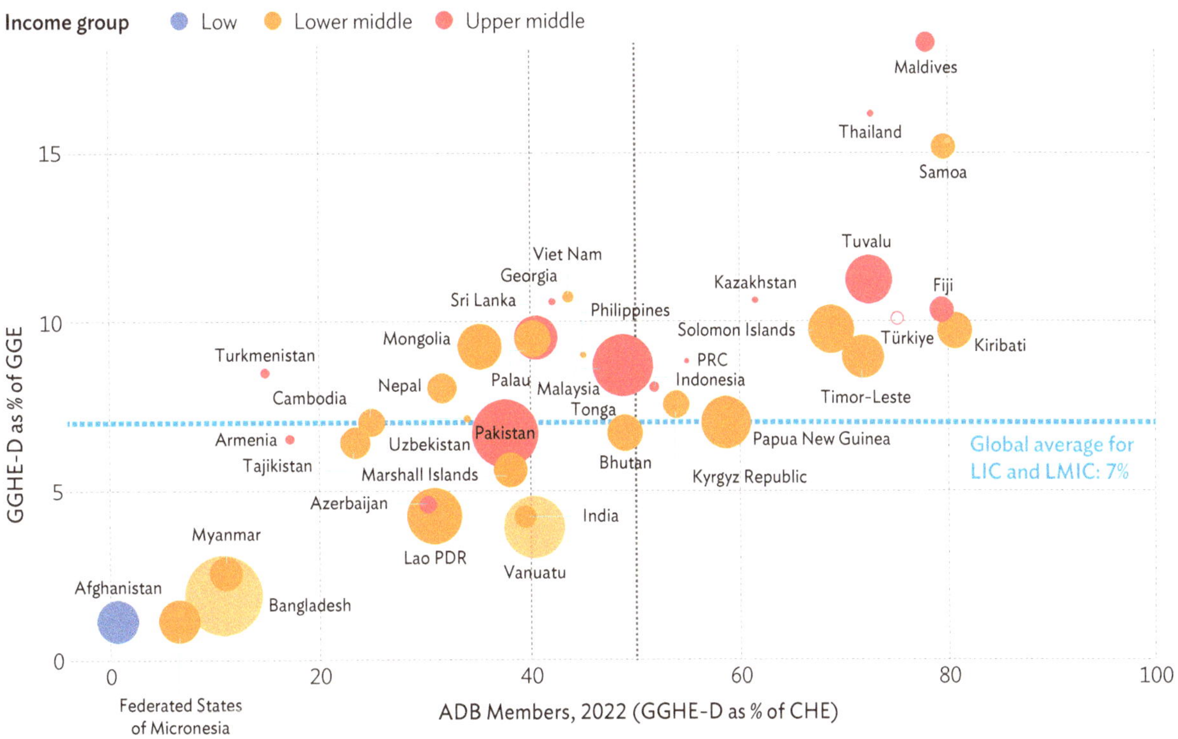

ADB = Asian Development Bank, CHE = current health expenditure, GGE = general government expenditure, GGHE-D = domestic general government health expenditure, Lao PDR = Lao People's Democratic Republic, LIC = low-income country, LMIC = low- and middle-income country, PRC = People's Republic of China.

Notes: (i) ADB placed its regular assistance to Afghanistan on hold effective 15 August 2021.
(ii) Effective 1 February 2021, ADB placed a temporary hold on sovereign project disbursements and new contracts in Myanmar.

Source: World Health Organization. 2024. Global Health Expenditure Database.

Box 7

Evolution in Health Taxes: The Case of the Philippines

According to the International Monetary Fund, lower- and middle-income countries have an untapped tax potential of up to 9 percentage points of gross domestic product, representing a significant opportunity to bolster domestic financing for health and pandemic prevention, preparedness, and response. Realizing this potential requires a dual strategy: (i) strengthening tax administration and enforcement to improve compliance and efficiency; and (ii) reforming tax policy, including broadening the tax base and introducing new instruments such as health taxes (e.g., on tobacco, alcohol, and sugary beverages), which can simultaneously promote public health and generate revenues. The Philippines has implemented a series of health tax reforms since 2012, notably through excise taxes on tobacco and vaping products, alcohol, and sugar-sweetened beverages. These reforms significantly increased government revenues, with tobacco excise tax collections rising from ₱32.9 billion in 2012 to ₱99.5 billion in 2015—a 202% increase. A substantial portion of these revenues was allocated for health, with 80% allocated to expanding access to the Philippine Health Insurance Corporation (PhilHealth) for low-income households and the remainder supporting broader health system strengthening.

Source: F. J. Chaloupka and L. Powell. 2019. *Health Taxes to Save Lives—Background Materials: Case Studies.* Prepared for the Task Force on Fiscal Policy for Health.

In six ADB DMCs (Bhutan, Indonesia, the Lao People's Democratic Republic, Mongolia, Pakistan, and Sri Lanka), external debt servicing represents more than 10% of general government expenditure. This dynamic not only limits fiscal flexibility but also risks entrenching cycles of underinvestment and dependence on external aid. Comprehensive debt management, restructuring, and relief are therefore essential—not only to restore fiscal sustainability but also to unlock budgetary space, specifically for PPPR, and more broadly for health (Box 7). However, fiscal space alone is not sufficient—political will and institutional capacity are equally important.

Strengthening public financing management for pandemic prevention, preparedness, and response

Requirements of an effective PPPR. Effective PPPR requires not only adequate financing but also the capacity to allocate, disburse, and monitor resources efficiently and accountably. This makes public financial management (PFM) systems a critical enabler of resilient and responsive health systems. To ensure countries can act swiftly during health emergencies, PFM systems must be proactively adapted during preparedness periods—well before a crisis strikes (Figure 7). Reforms are needed across all three stages of the budget cycle:

(1) *Budget formulation and allocation:* PPPR financing should be systematically integrated into national budgets, with clear allocations and contingency provisions. Mechanisms must allow for flexible reallocation across programs and funding sources, enabling governments to respond rapidly to evolving threats without waiting for supplementary appropriations.

(2) *Budget execution and disbursement:* In emergencies, delays in the release of funds can cost lives. PFM systems must be equipped to disburse funds quickly and flexibly—particularly to frontline service providers. This requires adjusting regulations during preparedness periods to enable decentralized spending authority, ensure liquidity at subnational levels, and streamline procurement processes.

(3) *Monitoring and accountability:* Transparent tracking of PPPR expenditures is essential to build public trust and ensure effective use of resources. Financial management information systems should be adapted to integrate emergency-related spending.

Figure 7: Agile Public Financial Management Systems to Enable Effective Health Emergency Response

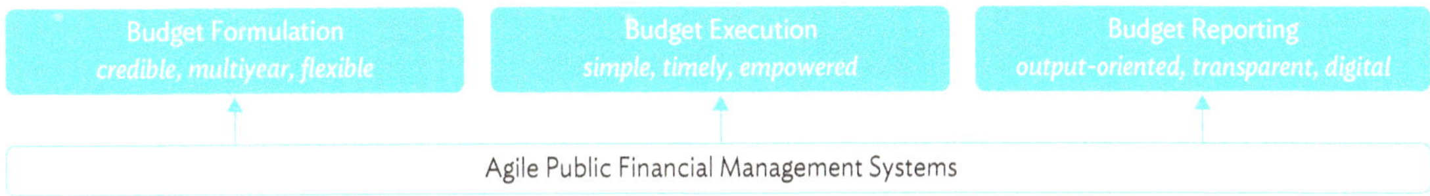
Budget Formulation
credible, multiyear, flexible
Budget Execution
simple, timely, empowered
Budget Reporting
output-oriented, transparent, digital
Agile Public Financial Management Systems

Source: World Health Organization. 2022. *Public Financial Management for Effective Response to Health Emergencies: Key Lessons from COVID-19 for Balancing Flexibility and Accountability*.

> Strong accountability and reporting mechanisms will help deter misuse of funds and inform future budget allocations.

New PPPR financing instruments—such as the Pandemic Fund and the International Monetary Fund's Resilience and Sustainability Facility[32]—are increasingly designed to support PFM reforms. Such instruments should continue to evolve in a way that permits countries to be in charge of their own preparedness planning; priorities, including for procurement, should not be bound to the priorities of competitive financing instruments. These instruments offer both financial incentives and capacity-building support to help countries modernize their PFM systems and embed PPPR priorities into core budgeting and monitoring processes (Box 8). Country PFM operations—such as those developed in Cambodia[33] or Maldives[34]—need to be cognizant of PPPR requirements and consider tailoring rules and processes to make PFM systems more responsive to crises and shocks. Well designed, they can provide a win–win, enhancing the volume and quality of PPPR financing, while reinforcing the institutional foundations for long-term health system resilience and ensuring gradual increases in national government funding.

Box 8

Leveraging the Resilience and Sustainability Facility for Pandemic Prevention, Preparedness, and Response-Related Public Financial Management and Governance Reforms—The Case of the Hashemite Kingdom of Jordan

The Hashemite Kingdom of Jordan's experience demonstrates how the International Monetary Fund's Resilience and Sustainability Facility (RSF) can be leveraged to accelerate public financial management and governance reforms that strengthen pandemic preparedness and response. In 2025, Jordan secured a 30-month RSF arrangement worth approximately $700 million to address vulnerabilities, including in the health sector. The RSF will serve as a catalytic instrument, aligning financial support with institutional reforms that bolster Jordan's capacity to respond to future health emergencies, and to sustain this capacity in the long term.

Source: World Health Organization. 2025. WHO Welcomes IMF Support to Jordan for Pandemic Preparedness and Response. News release. 4 July.

ADB's ongoing support for PFM strengthening (e.g., through policy-based lending and technical assistance) can play a catalytic role in advancing this agenda.[35]

32 International Monetary Fund. 2025. *Resilience and Sustainability Facility—Updated Operational Guidance Note*.

33 ADB. Cambodia: Strengthening Public Financial Management Program, Subprogram 1.

34 Government of the Philippines, Department of Budget and Management. 2025. *Public Financial Management Reforms Roadmap Now in Full Swing*. Press release. 14 May.

35 Independent Evaluation Department. 2021. *Addressing the COVID-19 Crisis: Lessons from Support for Public Financial Management*. Synthesis Note. No. 6. ADB.

Domestic funding is at the heart of pandemic prevention, preparedness, and response

Tracking pandemic prevention, preparedness, and response spending

PPPR—inherently multisector. PPPR encompasses health, animal health, environmental surveillance, and emergency response systems. Even within the health sector, PPPR spans a broad spectrum of activities—from targeted interventions addressing pandemic-prone pathogens to foundational investments in health system capacities such as surveillance, laboratory infrastructure, and workforce development. The workforce in primary care settings, for example, may split their time between routine individual prevention and health care, and prevention and detection activities. This complexity poses significant challenges for defining a universally accepted scope of PPPR spending, as well as to budget and track the financial resources. Ideally, expenditure data would comprehensively capture all relevant activities across sectors. In practice, however, data sources remain fragmented and methodologically inconsistent, making data aggregation across sectors unreliable. Within the health sector alone, accurate budgeting and monitoring is constrained by the limited production of National Health Accounts in many LMICs.

Tools used to assess country capacity under the IHR are an effective way of detecting and measuring gaps in PPPR efforts. However, they do not provide direct estimates of the investment required to improve such capacity, and must be supplemented with costing exercises, which, to date, have been sporadic. The lack of sufficiently detailed PPPR investment plans remains an obstacle for medium-term financial planning and accountability.

Addressing this gap calls for investments in digital infrastructure, the institutionalization of routine data collection, and the development of analytical capacities.[36] Embedding PPPR expenditure tracking within national financial management information systems is also critical. This would enable more systematic and routine monitoring of public spending on PPPR, support evidence-informed budget allocations, and contribute to building resilient, transparent, and accountable financing systems. At the regional and global levels, persistent tracking gaps highlighted by the High-Level Independent Panel also continue to limit visibility and coordination. Establishing a global tracker for PPPR and health financing would enhance transparency and accountability, build trust in public action, and inform strategic investment planning.

Scaling day-zero financing

Timing—decisive in pandemics. COVID-19 showed that the principal limitation was not scientific innovation but financing prior to and at the onset of the pandemic. Vaccines were developed in record time, yet access was not equitable because funds to secure vaccines and stimulate production at the scale needed were not available. COVAX, for example, took more than 15 months to raise $10 billion, by which point initial supplies had largely been reserved by countries that could pay up front. The result was predictable: delayed deliveries, deep inequities, and, arguably, a prolonged global recovery. Another cause for delay was the absence of national systems to vaccinate adults in countries where adult vaccination systems for diseases such as influenza are absent.[37] Country-by-country loans were slow to disburse and added debt burdens. Hybrid cost-sharing schemes required fiscal space that many governments lacked.

[36] WHO. 2024. National Health Accounts: Tracking Health Investments Towards Better Health for All. Feature story. 13 December.

[37] G. Gotsadze et al. 2023. Adult Vaccination in Asia and the Pacific: Policies, Financial Needs, and Fiscal Impacts. *ADB Sustainable Development Working Paper Series*. No. 90. ADB.

Donor pledges eventually enabled pooled procurement, but they came after the crucial first wave of production slots was already allocated. Late financing cannot secure early access.

The solution is day-zero financing: a pre-arranged, pooled liquidity line housed at multilateral development banks (MDBs) and backed by donors. Activation would be automatic once a pandemic threat is declared, enabling immediate advance purchase agreements for vaccines, tests, and treatments. This ensures that early access depends on readiness, not fiscal space. National resources can still fund delivery, but the initial bottleneck to access is removed. Modest prearranged commitments can prevent trillion-dollar delays and save lives (Box 9 and Box 10).

Box 9

Improving Financial Instruments and Frameworks for Pandemic Response —Lessons from the Inter-American Development Bank

Prearranged contingent financing instruments can offer quick liquidity to governments during health emergencies. Ideally, these instruments should incorporate features that proved essential during the coronavirus disease (COVID-19) pandemic, such as timeliness and flexibility. For instance, the Inter-American Development Bank (IDB) authorized the short-term use of their Contingent Credit Facility for COVID-19 Response but simultaneously reformed the instrument into a permanent modality for public health emergencies. This modality now offers up to 1% of gross domestic product or $100 million (whichever is lowest) in the event of a declared national health emergency and has been approved for Argentina, Bahamas, Bolivia, Colombia, Ecuador, El Salvador, Honduras, Panama, and Suriname.

Additional pre-pandemic financing options currently under consideration by the IDB include the following:

- **Deferred drawdown options:** These involve designing and approving loans during noncrisis periods for disbursement upon a preagreed trigger. Deferred drawdown options can be applied to both policy-based loans, which support reforms and public policy improvements; and investment loans, which fund infrastructure and service delivery. Both loan types could be used to procure medical countermeasures or strengthen health systems to better respond to pandemics.
- **Emergency component:** This is an optional feature within investment loans that allows flexible reallocation of funds between components, without a cap, enabling disbursements within weeks. Currently, only a limited percentage of investment loan budget can be transferred without Board approval. Key elements such as risk assessments, vulnerability levels, and activation triggers would be defined during the design phase.
- **Post-emergency financing:** Instruments designed and approved after a crisis has occurred are also under consideration as part of broader financial reforms.[a] A new instrument is under development to replace the Immediate Response Facility, aimed at supporting rapid disaster response and early reconstruction. Eligibility criteria and eligible expenditures would be defined during project design. Importantly, the instrument would offer full flexibility for retroactive financing, allowing countries to cover urgent expenses incurred prior to approval.
- **National adult vaccination systems:** COVID-19 showcased countries the importance of having mechanisms to deliver vaccines at scale to populations at risk, in this case adults. Many countries have limited or no routine adult vaccination programs necessitating comprehensive emergency vaccine deployment plans for all scenarios or institution of new adult vaccination programs.[b]

[a] At the time of writing this document, these proposals are yet to be submitted for consideration by the Executive Board.

[b] World Health Organization. 2024. National Health Accounts: Tracking Health Investments Towards Better Health for All. Feature story. 13 December.

Source: Inter-American Development Bank. 2025. Symposium on Multilateral Financing for Pandemic Preparedness. INSPIRE Health Forum. Manila.

Box 10

Enhancing Coherence of Pandemic Prevention, Preparedness, and Response Financing

The newly established **Coordinating Financing Mechanism**, under the amended International Health Regulations and the Pandemic Agreement, offers a critical platform to enhance coherence, predictability, and equity in global pandemic prevention, preparedness, and response financing. By aligning financial flows with national priorities and facilitating access to surge financing during emergencies, the mechanism aims to address long-standing challenges of fragmentation and inefficiency. Its success will depend on transparent governance, country ownership, and integration with broader sustainable financing strategies of the health sector.

The **World Bank's Crisis Preparedness and Response Toolkit** (CPRT), launched in 2024, represents a significant evolution in how international financial institutions integrate resilience into development finance. Rather than relying solely on ex-post emergency lending, the CPRT embeds prearranged crisis financing and debt-service flexibility directly into sovereign lending portfolios. Through instruments such as the Rapid Response Option and the Investment Project Financing Deferred Drawdown Option, countries can repurpose up to 10% of undisbursed funds or access contingent credit lines when emergencies strike. This accelerates response without new borrowing or prolonged approval processes. Complementary Climate-Resilient Debt Clauses allow temporary suspension of repayments following qualifying disasters, freeing fiscal space for urgent recovery needs.

The CPRT also advances an institutional model for preparedness. The Ready-to-Respond Diagnostic and the Crisis Preparedness Gap Analysis tools assess national readiness across governance, fiscal, and operational dimensions, helping governments identify bottlenecks and prioritize investments. These diagnostics have already been deployed in fragile and small-state contexts, guiding reforms in risk governance and budgetary resilience. Early applications in Mozambique and the Caribbean have demonstrated tangible benefits in the form of preagreed contingent funds and the Climate-Resilient Debt Clause activation enabled governments to mobilize resources within days of cyclones and hurricanes, reducing the lag between disaster onset and fiscal response. This exemplifies a shift from reactive crisis management to anticipatory resilience financing. By linking diagnostics, prearranged finance, and debt flexibility, the framework offers a replicable model for other multilateral development banks. For the Asia and Pacific region where disasters due to natural hazards, pandemics, and climate shocks increasingly intersect, adapting CPRT-like mechanisms within regional development portfolios could ensure liquidity, stability, and institutional readiness before crises escalate. It underscores how innovation by international finance institutions can convert financial instruments into strategic tools for long-term pandemic and climate preparedness.

Beyond adapting old financing instruments and designing new ones, **coordination across international financing institutions is crucial** to enable coherent and sufficient surge-financing. Coordination was mostly ad hoc during the coronavirus disease (COVID-19) pandemic but should ideally follow a predefined path, minimize duplication, and maximize complementarity. The G20/World Bank/World Health Organization Operational Playbook for Pandemic Response Financing is a reference on the financing options from international finance institutions available to countries across the pandemic cycle.

Sources: G20 Joint Finance and Health Taskforce. 2024. *G20/World Bank/World Health Organization Operational Playbook for Pandemic Response Financing*; World Bank. 2024. *Crisis Preparedness and Response: Best Practices and Lessons Learned from Contingent Emergency Response Component (CERC) Activations and Implementation;* and World Health Organization. 2025. *The WHO Pandemic Agreement.*

Utilizing innovative and blended financing approaches

Innovative and blended financing approaches—closing the investment gap in PPPR. The establishment of the Pandemic Fund represented a pivotal step in this direction, demonstrating how grant-based catalytic funding can mobilize additional resources from MDBs, bilateral donors, and domestic stakeholders. With a leverage ratio of approximately 1:7, the Pandemic Fund exemplifies how blended finance can crowd in concessional and domestic public resources to support country-led PPPR priorities.[38] To accelerate progress toward sustainable and self-reliant financing, there is a growing need to systematize the use of grant financing from global health initiatives—such as Gavi and the Global Fund—to catalyze MDB investments. This aligns with the recommendations of the High-Level Independent Panel, which called for dedicated concessional windows within MDBs and stronger partnerships with global health initiatives to enhance the resilience of health systems.[39]

Transitional financing offers a complementary, fit-for-purpose approach for countries advancing toward domestic financing.[40] Typically structured as time-bound grants blended with concessional loans, transitional financing can support institutional capacity building in areas such as PFM, surveillance, supply chains, or procurement. By embedding clear incentives and co-investment mechanisms, this model can enhance both fiscal sustainability and programmatic impact. This is especially important given the prevailing fiscal challenges faced by many economies and the lessons learned in sustaining services following loss of external grant financing.[41] Beyond traditional health sector tools, nontraditional financing instruments—such as guarantees, bonds, or debt swaps—can unlock new sources of capital. These efforts should be complemented by regional market-shaping strategies, including collaborative procurement and local manufacturing incentives, to attract foreign direct investment and strengthen regional supply chains.

Aligning aid with national systems

Inefficiencies in delivery of health aid. COVID-19 exposed critical inefficiencies in how official development assistance is delivered in the health sector. Fragmented aid flows—often routed through parallel systems and multiple implementing entities and budget holders—led to duplication, inconsistent responses, and an excessive reporting burden for recipient countries. These challenges, highlighted by the Independent Panel for Pandemic Preparedness and Response, underscore the urgent need to reevaluate how external resources are channeled and used.[42] To enhance the impact and sustainability of PPPR financing, a shift toward greater alignment with national systems is essential in keeping with principles outlined in the Lusaka Agenda (2023).[43]

38 ADB is one of the 13 implementing entities through which the Pandemic Fund channels its resources. These entities are responsible for administering funds, providing technical assistance, and supporting project implementation in recipient countries.

39 G20 High Level Independent Panel. 2025. *Closing the Deal: Financing Our Security Against Pandemic Threats*.

40 International Commission of Experts on Financing for Development. 2025. *Financing a Sustainable Future: Proposals for a Renewed Global Development Finance Agenda*.

41 M. Pincombe, P. Baker, A. Gheorghe, and J. Madan Keller. 2023. Projections of Eligibility and Transition Trajectories up to 2040: Implications for Gavi's Next Strategic Period and Beyond. *CGD Policy Papers*. No. 316. Center for Global Development.

42 E. Radin and C. Eleftheriades. 2021. *Financing Pandemic Preparedness and Response*. Background Paper 14. Commissioned by the Independent Panel for Pandemic Preparedness and Response.

43 Future of Global Health Initiatives. 2023. *The Lusaka Agenda: Conclusions of the Future of Global Health Initiatives Process*.

Financing Alignment Indicators

Budget Cycle Stage	Indicator	Rationale
Budget preparation	Donor funding for health included in annual budget as % of total donor funding for health	Shows transparency and alignment, as well as efficiency of donor funding with country budgeting systems
Budget execution	Donor funding for health spent through domestic expenditure management mechanism	Shows integration of donor funding into country expenditure management system (or use of parallel system)
	Donor funding for health disbursed to governments as % of total approved funding for health	Shows predictability of donor funding
	Donor funding for health disbursed accounted for through domestic financial management system	Shows integration of donor funding into country accounting and control systems
	Donor funding for health reported through domestic financial reporting system	Indicates level of alignment with country financial reporting procedures
Budget accountability	Donor funding for health audited through domestic auditing procedures	Indicates level of alignment with country auditing system

Source: S. Sparkes, H. Barroy, K. Chalkidou, P. Baker, and S. Witter. 2025. Money Talks: The Lusaka Agenda Financing Alignment Indicators. Blog post. Center for Global Development. 9 January.

This includes integrating external support into national health sector plans, budget cycles, and PFM systems. Doing so would not only strengthen country ownership and accountability but would also improve the efficiency and coherence of investments—particularly when PPPR financing contributes to broader health system strengthening. Such alignment also reduces transaction costs and fosters long-term institutional capacity. Tracking progress on this alignment agenda for the health sector is essential (see table on Financing Alignment Indicators).[44] While there is no formal regional equivalent to the Lusaka Agenda in Asia and the Pacific, its principles strongly resonate with the needs and priorities of this region, where fragmented aid delivery and parallel systems have long posed challenges to sustainable health financing.[45] These principles are reflected in ADB-supported initiatives such as The Pacific Approach 2021–2025,[46] ADB's regional strategy for Pacific developing member countries, which emphasizes country ownership, regional cooperation, and resilient service delivery systems.

Pandemic prevention, preparedness, and response investments reflect choices and trade-offs

[44] S. Sparkes, H. Barroy, K. Chalkidou, P. Baker, and S. Witter. 2025. Money Talks: The Lusaka Agenda Financing Alignment Indicators. Blog post. Center for Global Development. 9 January.

[45] P. Leka. 2025. Pacific Health Systems: Breaking the Aid Dependency Cycle. *The Interpreter* (Lowy Institute). 15 May.

[46] ADB. 2021. *Pacific Approach 2021–2025*.

GOVERNANCE GAPS AND OPPORTUNITIES

▶ Aligning mandates for more coherent governance and financing

PPPR global architecture—fragmented, with overlapping mandates and time-bound resources. The Pandemic Agreement and the amended IHR seek to formalize coordination through binding obligations on transparency, data sharing, and equitable access. Yet, financing also remains a constraint. Strengthening global governance will mean aligning mandates: WHO for norms and oversight; MDBs for financial sustainability; and regional entities such as ADB for country-level implementation and monitoring. Embedding preparedness within fiscal-sustainability frameworks including sovereign risk models, national development plans, and debt-relief mechanisms can reframe PPPR as an economic safeguard rather than an emergency cost.

▶ Supporting community-centered governance

Community-level crisis management. Public health crises are not navigated solely in ministries and hospitals, but also in communities. A truly resilient system empowers communities as partners in governance, not just recipients of policy. Crucially, these systems facilitate two-way communications—from village concerns to national policy and back again—with accountability and transparent metrics that bridge the complexity of health systems with the understanding of communities. Resolve to Save Lives' 7-1-7 target,[47] which involves finding suspected outbreaks within 7 days, reporting to public health authorities within 1 day, and mounting an effective response within 7 days, offers a clear, measurable, and achievable goal. When countries openly and regularly share their performance against such metrics, they not only strengthen public understanding and interest in public health but also provide a tangible measure of government effectiveness in detecting and responding to threats. During COVID-19, delays in disseminating critical information eroded public confidence; by contrast, sharing metrics like 7-1-7, alongside alert thresholds that communicate the level of risk and steps to be taken by individuals and communities, create a common language for action. It supports governance across sectors and builds trust between institutions and the people they serve (Box 11).

Box 11

Rethinking Governance Models to Manage Trade-Offs, Not Avoid Them

Investing in health security through financing preparedness is a highly cost-effective way to protect lives, safeguard livelihoods and communities, and ensure the stability of governance and governments. Whether measured in human lives saved or economic disruption avoided, the return on investment for pandemic preparedness is extraordinarily high. To make this possible, the financial ecosystem that supports governance must adopt three key strategies:

1. **Funding preparedness as core infrastructure:** Pandemic preparedness and response systems must be built into public institutions, not treated as an add-on emergency expense. They must be regarded as core institutional infrastructure, not merely as a reactive response to be activated only during times of crises. Development banks must mainstream this funding across all sectors—housing, education, urban planning—because all are implicated in public health resilience.

continued on next page

[47] Resolve to Save Lives. 7-1-7: A Global Target for Early Detection and Response.

Box 11 *continued*

2. **Measuring what truly matters:** Metrics should capture trust, cross-sector coordination, and community participation—not just hospital bed capacity. Development finance institutions should invest in new metrics and monitoring systems that capture functional capabilities, trust, coordination, and inclusion. These indicators should inform loan conditionalities and investment priorities, as well as improve tracking.
3. **Designing systems for trade-offs:** Decision-making must be built to navigate complexity, not to obscure it. Governments must transparently balance saving lives, protecting economies, and preserving social bonds, and explain those choices clearly to the people who will live with their consequences. Transparent, participatory governance models must be funded and embedded into public institutions. Development banks should support tools like alert frameworks, real-time dashboards, and deliberative public forums that help manage the inherent tensions in crisis decision-making.

By framing preparedness as a driver of social stability, economic continuity, and political legitimacy, development banks can shift the narrative from cost to value. Multilateral development banks are uniquely positioned to catalyze cross-sector collaboration and drive systemic change by supporting institutions that can manage complexity with agility and equity, making the case—rigorously and repeatedly—that investing in pandemic governance is investing in every other sector they care about.

Source: Resolve to Save Lives. 2025. Symposium on Multilateral Financing for Pandemic Preparedness. INSPIRE Health Forum. Manila.

Development banks can reinforce this participatory model by requiring community engagement as a condition for funding and by directly supporting subnational governance capacity. Moreover, they can help create feedback mechanisms that allow communities to influence how preparedness programs are designed, financed, and evaluated—strengthening democratic accountability in the process (Box 12).

Box 12

Governance Case Studies

Case Study 1: Republic of Korea's Governance and Public Health Infrastructure

A critical element of the successful response to the coronavirus disease (COVID-19) pandemic in the Republic of Korea was the whole-of-government approach that included well-defined governance structures and seamless cooperation among different ministries, and between central and local authorities.

1. **Coordination and command structure:** The Republic of Korea's COVID-19 response was directed by a clear, predefined, and centralized command structure under the Prime Minister, who led the Central Disaster and Safety Countermeasure Headquarters for a swift, whole-of-government approach. Under this unified command, the Korea Center for Disease Control managed the technical public health response, the Ministry of Health and Welfare oversaw the health care system, and the Ministry of Interior and Safety coordinated broad societal and administrative support.
2. **Cooperation with local governments:** The central body coordinated with the Local Disaster and Safety Countermeasure Headquarters and the local disease control task forces established in every province and major city, ensuring that national strategies were implemented effectively at the community level.
3. **Risk communication:** The government prioritized prompt and transparent communication. Daily briefings were held to update the public, and emergency alerts were used to disseminate information about local outbreaks, reinforcing adherence to public health guidelines.

continued on next page

Box 12 *continued*

Case Study 2: Transparent, Adaptive Governance in Action from Resolve to Save Lives

The experience of **Thailand's Samut Sakhon Province** illustrates the value of **targeted, localized, and adaptive responses**, demonstrating what can happen when governments move beyond limiting siloed thinking and adopt a more comprehensive systems approach. Instead of imposing costly blanket lockdowns during COVID-19, Samut Sakhon authorities used real-time surveillance data to identify hot spots and target interventions—especially among migrant workers in seafood markets—and thus were able to maintain economic activity. They also deployed mobile testing, localized isolation and quarantines, and community health volunteers, while ensuring food provision and social support. This localized, data-driven approach was only possible through preexisting public health infrastructure and effective governance coordination, and exemplifies how governments can manage competing priorities with agility and fairness.

To make balanced policy decisions, weighing health impact against secondary effects of public health and social measures requires good governance and reliable data. During COVID-19, the Partnership for Evidence-Based Response to COVID-19 initiative worked with **20 African governments to build multisector data platforms**. These data ecosystems informed more nuanced decision-making, allowing leaders to help find the balance of slowing transmission while minimizing secondary impacts. This data system facilitated not only evaluation of viral spread but also weighing of epidemiologic trends against social and economic pressures in real time, thereby enabling informed, transparent, and explainable decisions that are grounded in the social contract between the government and its citizens.

Ghana used real-time data on transmission, economic impact, and social stress to adjust restrictions on a neighborhood-by-neighborhood basis. When cases spiked in the markets of the densely populated capital, Accra, government officials did not shut down the whole city—they increased testing and support in those specific areas while keeping schools and other sectors open.

Crucially, the emphasis here is not just on technical sophistication but on **transparent governance**. In other examples, countries that adopted **alert-level systems frameworks—such as New Zealand, Singapore, and South Africa**—were able to provide the public with predefined alert thresholds and corresponding actions to be taken at each level. This clarity fostered trust and predictability, using clear alert levels, predefined triggers, and public communication to help governments act early and help people understand what would happen next and why transmission levels increased.

Such initiatives should not be treated as crisis-specific projects, but as scalable models for institutional reform. Multilateral development banks are uniquely placed to support these efforts through long-term technical assistance, concessional financing, and results-based investment instruments that reward governance innovation and resilience.

Sources: Hoon Sang Lee, the RIGHT Foundation. 2025. Symposium on Multilateral Financing for Pandemic Preparedness. INSPIRE Health Forum. Manila; and Amanda McClelland, Resolve to Save Lives. 2025. Symposium on Multilateral Financing for Pandemic Preparedness. INSPIRE Health Forum. Manila.

Creating an Operational Ecosystem for Equitable Access to Vaccines, Therapeutics, and Diagnostics

Learning health systems are better positioned to adapt during crises

RESEARCH AND DEVELOPMENT GAPS AND OPPORTUNITIES

▶ **Investing in research and development**

COVID-19, demonstrated what science can achieve under pressure. Within a year, multiple effective vaccines were developed and deployed—an unprecedented achievement compared to the 4 years it took to produce the mumps vaccine, or the decades with no vaccines for pathogens such as malaria or Ebola. Behind this breakthrough was an extraordinary surge in research: by April 2020, as many new clinical trials had been launched for COVID-19 as for all other diseases combined, and by year's end more than 200 vaccine candidates were in the pipeline. Estimates indicate that research and development (R&D) activity during COVID-19 was **4 to 26 times larger** than expected given the market size—evidence that early public support and incentives helped unlock a surge of innovation. Importantly, public institutions accounted for about 70% of clinical trials, underscoring the role of government, universities, and hospitals in driving discovery.[48] While pharmaceutical innovation can be scaled up far more than previously assumed, this is contingent on sustained investment and incentives. Public support should extend not just to early-stage research but also to technology transfer and equitable diffusion of knowledge.

Upgrading the global R&D tool kit through, for example, universal coronavirus vaccines, novel antivirals, and stronger genomic surveillance, will be critical. To maximize impact, regions like Asia and the Pacific, Africa, and Latin America need greater participation in this innovation ecosystem, with financing to support discovery, clinical trials, and regulatory capacity. This necessitates collaboration between donors as no single donor supports product development and implementation through all stages—a nascent approach for Asia, the **Asian Coalition for Financing Research, Vaccine Development and Other Innovations**, has been agreed on by ADB, Global Health Innovative Technology Fund, RIGHT Foundation, SEA DREAM, and Temasek Foundation (Figure 8).

Equity in access to medical countermeasures is a global public good

MANUFACTURING GAPS AND OPPORTUNITIES

▶ **Strengthening regional manufacturing of vaccines, therapeutics, and diagnostics and other tools**

Concentrated manufacturing and fragmented procurement. Ten economies still control more than 80% of global vaccine R&D and production.[49] The global community is converging on the need for regional manufacturing ecosystems supported by technology transfer and collaborative procurement to achieve more equitable vaccine production and distribution (Box 13 and Box 14). Complementary investments in cold-chain resilience, digital logistics, and regulatory harmonization (e.g., participation in the WHO Listed Authority network) are essential for realizing these goals.

[48] R. Agarwal and P. Gaule. 2022. What Drives Innovation? Lessons from COVID-19 R&D. *Journal of Health Economics*. 82. 102591.

[49] WHO. 2023. *Global Vaccine Market Report: 2023 Update*.

Figure 8: End-to-End Funding of the Development and Introduction of Vaccines, Therapeutics, and Diagnostics Through Joined-Up Financing of Donors Active in Asia

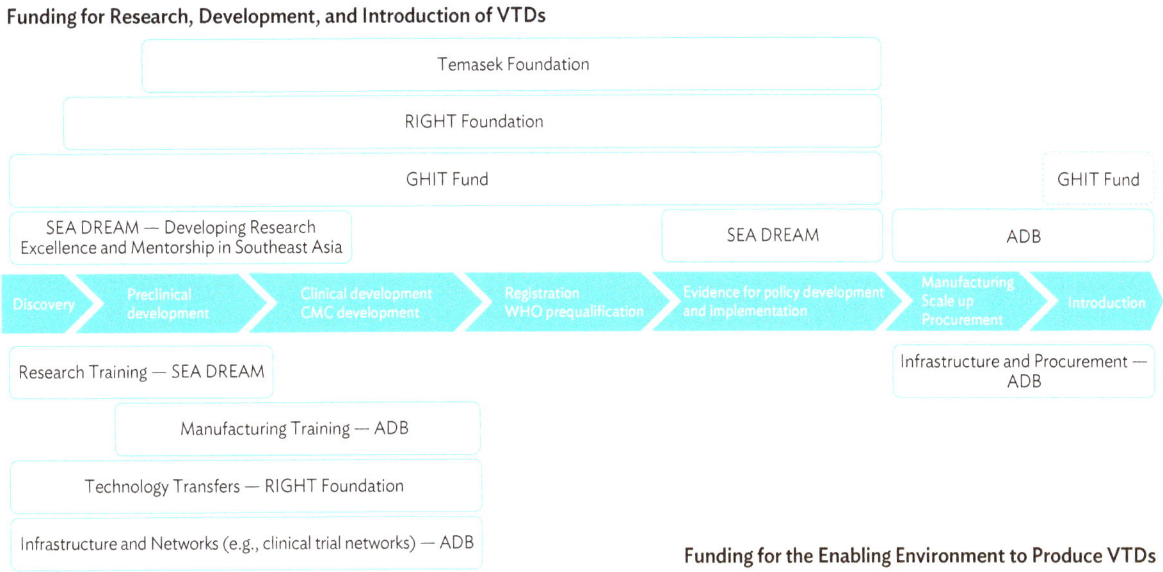

ADB = Asian Development Bank; CMC = chemistry, manufacturing, and controls; GHIT = Global Health Innovative Technology; RIGHT = Research Investment for Global Health Technology; VTD = vaccines, therapeutics, and diagnostics; RIGHT = Research Investment for Global Health Technology; WHO = World Health Organization.

Source: Asian Coalition for Financing Research, Vaccine Development, and Other Innovations.

This would result in enormous economic benefits: reducing the time from pathogen identification to vaccine availability from 9 months to 3 months could save $2 trillion–$3 trillion in global output losses in a severe pandemic.[50] The 100-Day Mission of the Coalition for Epidemic Preparedness Innovation (CEPI) and WHO's mRNA Vaccine Technology-Transfer Hub (South Africa) are prototypes in this direction. Similar initiatives in Asia, such as the ASEAN Vaccine Security and Self-Reliance Initiative, the Quad Vaccine Partnership, and India's expansion of bulk-antigen capacity can collectively shift the region from dependency to self-sufficiency.

[50] CEPI. The 100 Days Mission; and *McKinsey & Company*. 2024. Beyond the Pandemic: The Next Chapter of Innovation in Vaccines. 16 May.

Box 13

The Regionalized Vaccine Manufacturing Collaborative

The Regionalized Vaccine Manufacturing Collaborative (RVMC) promotes vaccine equity and security by establishing regional vaccine manufacturing and supply chain networks for routine and outbreak use that become part of the global ecosystem. In its latest report, RVMC emphasizes the need to address three key priorities for sustainable regional vaccine manufacturing:

1. More predictable demand and regional markets through mechanisms such as collaborative procurement;
2. Stronger regulatory systems and harmonization to accelerate approval and maintain quality; and
3. Further investments in integrated regional systems to link production, regulation, and demand across countries.

Source: RVMC. 2025. *Towards Regionalised Vaccine Manufacturing*. First Status Report.

Box 14

Beyond COVID-19: Manufacturing and Procurement Insights from H1N1, SARS, H5N1, and MERS

The swine flu (H1N1) pandemic in 2009 had a rapid vaccine rollout, with global vaccine companies developing H1N1 vaccines within months using existing flu vaccine technology. In Asia, some countries leveraged domestic vaccine capacity; others relied on global suppliers; and some, such as Japan and the Republic of Korea, used both. At least 10 People's Republic of China (PRC) manufacturers were mobilized to produce H1N1 vaccine doses, with 90 million doses manufactured and administered in less than 6 months. Indian firms, which initially lacked domestic flu vaccine production, quickly pivoted to become leading suppliers of H1N1 vaccines.

For the 2005 avian influenza (H5N1) pandemic, antiviral drugs rather than vaccines were the principal medical countermeasure. Countries around the world raced to stockpile Oseltamivir (Tamiflu). Governments, including in Asia, ordered millions of Tamiflu doses. Roche (Tamiflu's manufacturer) worked to enhance its supply; in late 2005, to meet overwhelming demand, it agreed to license production of Tamiflu to generic manufacturers, many based in India and the PRC. This experience underscores how technology transfer, when pursued in partnership with originator companies, can accelerate local readiness.

Severe acute respiratory syndrome (SARS) and Middle East respiratory syndrome (MERS) were less about vaccines and therapeutics and more about diagnostics. In Asia, these novel infections catalyzed investments in molecular diagnostic capacity, rapid diagnostic test development, and manufacturing. SARS, MERS, H5N1 (2005), and H1N1 (2009) all contributed to strengthened rapid test production for Japan's Fujirebio and the Republic of Korea's SD Biosensor. Protocols for the use of polymerase chain reaction tests by India's National Institute of Virology and in the PRC induced private manufacturers to start new diagnostic manufacturing, including Wondfo and BGI. In some ways, these were the foundational investments for the larger-scale coronavirus disease (COVID-19) test production that came later.

These four outbreaks reinforce the importance of regional and local production capacity in ensuring timely access to vaccines, therapeutics, and diagnostics at scale. They also provide several additional procurement lessons:

- **Stockpiling is sometimes essential, but the procurement required to maintain them is complex:** The H5N1 pandemic revealed the need for strategic stockpiles; yet, building and maintaining stockpiles, whether physical (finished product) or virtual (held in bulk by producers for later packaging) require forward-looking procurement strategies, financing mechanisms, and agreements with manufacturers to ensure supplies do not expire nor sit idle.
- **Preparedness must include antivirals and therapeutics, not just vaccines:** Vaccines are transformative for infections that can be prevented by them. But other tools matter in the early and mid-stages of pandemics, and if vaccine development is delayed or not feasible. Oseltamivir stockpiles, for example, shaped the H5N1 response, and monoclonal antibodies or oral antivirals may be central in future outbreaks.

Sources: A. Adbi, C. Chatterjee, and A. Mishra. 2022. How Do MNEs and Domestic Firms Respond Locally to a Global Demand Shock? Evidence from a Pandemic. *Management Science*. 68 (12). pp. 9003–9025; X. F. Liang et al. 2011. Safety of Influenza A (H1N1) Vaccine in Postmarketing Surveillance in China. *New England Journal of Medicine*. 364 (5). pp. 638–647; N. Watson, L. R. Kopczak, and P. Yadav. 2009. *When Supply Is of Public Interest: Roche & Tamiflu*. Harvard Business School Case Study; P. Yadav and A. Desir. 2021. *Boosting Vaccine Production Needs the Right Degree of Flexibility*. INSEAD Knowledge; and P. Yadav. 2025. Symposium on Multilateral Financing for Pandemic Preparedness. INSPIRE Health Forum. Manila.

ADB in Action 2

Procuring and Delivering Pandemic Vaccines—Challenges and Lessons Learned

The Asian Development Bank (ADB) established the Asia Pacific Vaccine Access Facility (APVAX) to finance coronavirus disease (COVID-19) vaccines for developing member countries (DMCs). The eligibility criteria for vaccines, however, posed challenges to timely procurement. As ADB does not have expertise in vaccine and medical product regulation, the criteria for financing COVID-19 vaccines relied on the regulatory approaches of the World Health Organization (WHO) and stringent regulatory authorities (SRAs)—vaccines had to meet at least one of the following criteria: (i) be selected for procurement through COVID-19 Vaccines Global Access (COVAX); (ii) receive WHO prequalification or emergency use listing; or (iii) gain authorization from a recognized SRA. Vaccines such as Pfizer-BNT, Moderna, AstraZeneca, and Johnson & Johnson gained regulatory approval in early 2021. However, WHO authorizations for Covishield, Sinopharm, Sinovac, Covaxin, and Novavax only came much later in 2021, with DMCs unable to utilize APVAX to purchase these vaccines. While criteria aimed to ensure vaccine procurement were in line with international best practices, many countries in the region were effectively blocked from accessing vaccines because of supply constraints arising from the advanced orders from high-income countries of vaccines that were approved earlier, and DMCs' limited fiscal capacity to make their own advance orders.

One lesson for ADB was that the approach did not consider where vaccines were being manufactured. Given the scale of the demand for vaccines, many were produced in new manufacturing facilities that had not been assessed by SRAs and, therefore, did not immediately qualify for purchasing through APVAX. Having clarity on regulatory requirements, and the importance of investing in regulatory systems across ADB members, are now known to be necessary for assuring supply of vaccines, therapeutics, and diagnostics (VTDs) during emergencies. At the same time, the WHO system of prequalification of vaccines should be reexamined to ensure that it is not a stumbling block to innovation and vaccine research and development in countries where risk benefit differs from that in the major vaccine-producing nations. As a result of these learnings, ADB has since launched two technical assistance projects (see ADB in Action 1)—(i) Asia Diagnostics, Vaccines, and Therapeutics Network to Counter Epidemics (**ADVaNCE**); and (ii) Strengthening Regulatory Ecosystem and Manufacturing for Vaccines, Therapeutics, and Diagnostics in Asia and the Pacific (**REVITALIZE**)—to strengthen DMC's national regulators, promote regulatory harmonization and convergence, develop mechanisms for collaborative procurement of VTDs, and support expansion of local and regional production capacity.

Source: ADB. 2025. Symposium on Multilateral Financing for Pandemic Preparedness. INSPIRE Health Forum. Manila.

REGULATORY GAPS AND OPPORTUNITIES

▶ Strengthening regulatory capacity

Regulatory standards and transferring technologies for vaccines, therapeutics, and diagnostics. The WHO process to recognize high performing national regulators (WHO-listed authorities)[51] is proceeding deliberately but slowly and WHO prequalification of many COVID-19 vaccines was protracted.

Developing regulatory preparedness, therefore, requires immediate investments in strengthening regulatory capacities in countries themselves, as well as driving regional regulatory coherence through mutual recognition agreements and fast-track approval mechanisms. Without strong national regulatory systems, VTDs cannot be authorized, tested, or deployed in a timely manner. Investing in regulatory ecosystems would not only strengthen VTD preparedness but also contribute to broader health system resilience (Box 15).

[51] WHO. WHO-Listed Authority (WLA).

ADB in Action 3

Regional Vaccine Advisory Group: Enabling Informed Vaccine Financing and Access

In June 2021, the **Regional Vaccine Advisory Group** was established to advise both the Asian Development Bank and its developing member countries on financing and purchasing of coronavirus disease (COVID-19) vaccines. This brought together national regulatory authorities, global health experts, and scientists from North America, the United Kingdom, and countries throughout Asia and the Pacific to expand vaccine access in the region through expert policy advice and sharing of regulatory approaches, and technical and scientific knowledge.

Source: Asian Development Bank.

Specific actions include the following:

- Capacity building for regulatory authorities, with a focus on good manufacturing practice inspections, lot release testing, and pharmacovigilance.
- Creating regional collaborative scientific forums (e.g., an Institute for Regulatory Science) for regulators to enable routine and rapid data sharing and peer review of dossiers during emergencies. ASEAN has precedents that can be drawn by other subregions.
- Encouraging reliance models, where smaller regulatory authorities in the region can rely on the decisions of larger, better resourced regulators, and can reduce duplication and speed up approvals.
- Assessing the suitability of the WHO prequalification scheme in the Asian region as it pertains to risk benefit of licensing VTDs developed in the region (and any adverse impacts on VTD innovation, research, and development).

Box 15

Enhancing the Asian Development Bank's Regulatory Advisory Services

In addition to regulatory capacity building, the Asian Development Bank (ADB) should consider convening a standing (or rapidly convened) *Regional Technical Advisory Panel on Pandemic Technologies*, a panel of independent regional technical experts, who, in close collaboration with national regulators, will advise on the potential risks and benefits of pandemic technologies that are not yet World Health Organization (WHO)-prequalified or approved by a WHO-listed authority. The panel could be called on to conduct expedited yet rigorous assessments of such technologies, evaluating their potential benefits and risks. It would advise ADB on when risk-mitigation measures and conditional approvals are necessary, such as requirements for post-marketing surveillance and ongoing performance data, and on the conduct of pharmacovigilance and other safety studies. The panel could also recommend fiscal measures to enhance research and development of critical vaccines, therapeutics, and diagnostics technologies and products in the region.

Source: P. Yadav. 2025. Symposium on Multilateral Financing for Pandemic Preparedness. INSPIRE Health Forum. Manila.

DELIVERY GAPS AND OPPORTUNITIES

Retooling procurement to share risk and incentivize readiness

Strategic procurement. Procurement is not simply a transactional and compliance-driven function; rather it is a strategic lever to share risk and incentivize supplier readiness for PPPR, and ultimately universal health coverage (UHC), ensuring that all people have access to the health products and services (e.g., vaccines and immunization) they need. For VTDs, this means moving beyond one-off contracts and creating structured arrangements that encourage manufacturers to maintain surge capacity, invest in adaptable platforms, and be willing to pivot quickly in the event of an outbreak. Some of these practices are already emerging in ADB's work, but require further institutionalization to ensure consistency, sustainability, and impact. Suppliers cannot be expected to build and maintain VTD capacity in isolation; instead, they need to integrate pandemic preparedness into their broader product portfolios. MDBs, including ADB, should systematically map and analyze these portfolios: What do manufacturers in the region produce today? How do their existing platforms align with potential pandemic technologies? What are their commercial incentives for prioritizing one product over another? How are these incentives related to advancing UHC?

Manufacturers' decisions on which products to manufacture are not driven solely by revenue potential. They also consider other factors, such as the following:

- **Lives saved and disability-adjusted life years averted**, particularly where donor support aligns with public health outcomes;
- **Platform familiarity**, as manufacturers prefer to work with technologies they already understand;
- **Donor and government interest**, which signals the likelihood of long-term market sustainability; and
- **Risk of failure and public scrutiny**, which may discourage investment in high-risk but high-need areas.

Procurement strategies must seek to influence these factors. This could be done through smart contract designs that reward early delivery and flexibility, and mechanisms that reduce reputational risks for suppliers taking on uncertain technologies. Traditional procurement relationships resemble a butterfly model: a narrow set of transactional connections between buyer and supplier, limited to tendering, and contract negotiation with only the supplier's sales team.[52] In a pandemic context (but also more generally), this approach is insufficient. A diamond model of engagement—characterized by multiple points of connection across operations, planning, finance, regulatory affairs, and supply chain logistics—offers multilayered relationships that could enable faster responses, improve demand forecasting and regulatory acceleration, and enhance mutual accountability. Admittedly, public sector transparency and accountability conditions require that deeper supplier relationships do not compromise fairness or open competition. This will require building systems of engagement that are not only strategic but also compliant.

Designing analytics for at-risk procurement portfolios

Early access to vaccines, therapeutics, and diagnostics. While the efforts of organizations such as CEPI[53] to maintain prototype repositories and ready-to-adapt platforms are notable and valuable, the reality is that, in almost all cases, no fully authorized VTDs will be available when the next pandemic begins.

52 Y. Wang and P. Yadav. 2005. *Strategic Procurement Outsourcing Assessment of Direct Material at Lucent EMEA*. MIT-Zaragoza International Program.

53 CEPI has been a global leader in investments to develop new pandemic vaccines and therapeutics.

Instead, multiple candidate technologies will still be in development, as was the case during COVID-19. In such a scenario, timely access depends on whether governments or their financiers, including MDBs, are willing to make advance purchase commitments "at risk" (i.e., committing funds before a product or technology has been authorized for use). Without such commitments, countries will inevitably find themselves at the back of the queue once a promising technology does succeed. This presents a dilemma: putting public money or MDB resources into a single unproven technology or a portfolio of technologies is a political and financial gamble, one that only industrialized countries were willing to take during the COVID-19 pandemic.

To navigate this challenge, clear processes and decision-making systems for at-risk procurement must be established. One promising approach is the use of simulation and portfolio modeling tools that estimate the probability of success for different technologies and their potential for rapid scale-up to help identify an "optimal subset" of candidates for advance purchase. This was precisely the logic behind the portfolio of vaccine advance purchase agreements by initiatives such as Operation Warp Speed in the United States and CEPI's COVID-19 portfolio (later embedded in COVAX). The Center for Global Development developed a modeling framework in April 2020 to estimate probabilities of success and projected manufacturing capacity for all COVID-19 vaccine candidates then under development.[54] Their analysis guided thinking about how to build resilient vaccine portfolios and assessed the choices made by Operation Warp Speed, CEPI, and other countries such as the United Kingdom.

This kind of modeling-plus-simulation approach could be institutionalized by MDBs to provide a standing capability to quickly evaluate evolving pipelines during a health emergency and deploy financing into the most promising subset of technologies. This would reduce delays, increase the efficiency of risk-taking, and improve vaccine equity. However, the legal, contractual, and governance implications of at-risk contracts remain complex. Issues such as liability, allocation of doses across countries, and enforceability of supply contracts need to be addressed up front. These challenges are precisely the reason why MDBs, such as ADB, in partnership country governments, should begin building frameworks now so that at-risk procurement decisions can be made with speed, rigor, and legitimacy when they are needed (Box 16).

A structured partnership with CEPI to tap into this expertise might include the following activities:

- Collaborating with CEPI on **portfolio modeling**, leveraging CEPI's experience in new pandemic technologies and manufacturing technology platforms, and their understanding of supplier portfolios;
- Conducting joint **table-top simulation exercises**, ensuring that MDB (and DMC) procurement and financing teams are prepared to make at-risk commitments under real-world scenarios; and
- Ensuring **greater flexibility in production assets** is essential, requiring investment in modular plants and adaptable platforms that enable rapid product switches. Because private manufacturers are unlikely to make such costly, uncertain investments alone, IFIs can utilize their financing, conditionality, and technical support to ensure the new emerging manufacturers in DMCs are embedding sufficient flexibility into their facility design and capital decisions. It can collaborate with CEPI to play the technical role in this regard.

[54] A. McDonnell et al. 2020. COVID-19 Vaccine Predictions: Using Mathematical Modelling and Expert Opinions to Estimate Timelines and Probabilities of Success of COVID-19 Vaccines. *CGD Policy Paper*. No. 183. Center for Global Development.

Box 16

Procurement as a Strategic Lever for Pandemic Preparedness

Under normal conditions, public procurement of vaccines, therapeutics, and diagnostics (VTDs) is designed to balance efficiency and cost-effectiveness with the ability to withstand public scrutiny, making it inherently a risk-averse (and compliance-focused) approach. “Strategic” procurement for the health sector has sought to broaden what public procurement can achieve through purchasing of routine products by managing market dynamics, fostering sustainable supply, and stimulating innovation. Three pillars have been fundamental to this approach:

1. **Demand aggregation and streamlined processes**—to obtain lower prices and expanded access;
2. **Healthy markets**—ensuring long-term viability by supporting a diverse supplier base and creating incentives for innovation; and
3. **A value chain perspective**—taking an end-to-end view that includes research and development, manufacturing, and last-mile delivery, rather than focusing narrowly on the most efficient way of buying finished products.

Procurement of emergency VTDs, however, has complexities beyond routine products. Their development cycles are uncertain, but can move very fast; surges in demand are unpredictable; and the urgency of their delivery is unmatched, since delays in securing VTDs can translate directly into large case burdens and lives lost. There is, therefore, a fundamental tension between health procurement systems’ traditional focus on risk minimization and the paramount need for speed and flexibility during a crisis—this puts procurement at the heart of pandemic preparedness and requires new capabilities on top of traditional skills. These include the following:

1. **Procurement at risk**—committing to purchases before full regulatory approval, a practice that was critical during the coronavirus disease (COVID-19) vaccine rollouts;
2. **Faster procurement cycles**—adapting processes so that speed consistently outweighs perfection when lives are at stake; and
3. **Supplier engagement**—developing a deep understanding of global markets, regional supply bases, and the entire product portfolios of individual suppliers, recognizing that many produce multiple critical items simultaneously, which means prioritization and portfolio fit are essential.

Equally important, procurement for VTDs must be aligned with regional regulatory pathways (Box 14). For smaller countries or those without domestic manufacturing, pooling procurement functions with other countries is not just about efficiency but may be the only pathway for timely access. The Asian Development Bank’s Asia Pacific Vaccine Access Facility (APVAX) has made it abundantly clear that financing, regulation, procurement, and supply chains must work in tandem to get VTDs from labs to populations at the pace demanded by health emergencies (ADB in Action 2).

Source: Prashant Yadav. 2025. Symposium on Multilateral Financing for Pandemic Preparedness. INSPIRE Health Forum. Manila.

Piloting regional collaborative procurement mechanisms in select subregions

For countries with small populations, collaborative procurement can yield significant benefits. These include (i) better pricing and supply terms for low-demand products that individual countries struggle to procure competitively; (ii) a foundation for regional solidarity and coordination, which can later be leveraged during health emergencies; and (iii) a platform for emergency response, where existing procurement systems can be quickly repurposed to secure pandemic VTDs. Collaborative procurement efforts require clear incentives for the participating parties (Box 17).

Box 17

Multilateral Procurement Platforms: COVID-19 Lessons from The Global Fund, COVAX, and Pan-American Health Organization's Revolving Fund

The Global Fund leveraged its pooled procurement mechanism for HIV, tuberculosis, and malaria for the coronavirus disease (COVID-19) pandemic countermeasures, personal protective equipment, and oxygen. Quality control was impacted by lockdowns and reduced regulatory capacity, while procurement challenges included limited demand visibility, delayed guidance, issues with mobilizing funds, and inequitable product allocation. Lessons for the future include timely issuance of clinical guidelines, leveraging partner networks, strengthening global coordination, mobilizing funding early, promoting transparency for low- and middle-income countries (LMICs), and accelerating regulatory harmonization. A standing global procurement coordination mechanism is critical for sustainable investment, country commitment, accountability, and transparency. The Global Fund's expertise and infrastructure position it as a key contributor to such an initiative.

COVAX (COVID-19 Vaccines Global Access) was a groundbreaking global initiative launched in 2020 to accelerate the development, manufacturing, and equitable access of COVID-19 vaccines. Resources were mobilized quickly through the platform, which was joined by more than 180 countries. After 1 year, the platform saw the first doses deployed to LMICs; after 2 years, more than 1 billion doses were delivered. Several of the vaccine candidates were effective, illustrating the importance of risk sharing. Despite the successes, the platform did not have enough financing to take risks or make better deals. Moreover, the diversification of production required and the lack of transparency were unexpected challenges. The global, instead of regional, focus of the platform was an additional challenge. One of the key lessons from COVAX was the need for regional and national procurement structures, combined with an awareness of supply chains, as no single country is likely to have all the components needed for a final vaccine product.

For over 40 years, the **Revolving Fund for Access to Vaccines of the Pan-American Health Organization** has ensured that countries can transparently purchase safe and quality-controlled vaccines at a negotiated, favorable price. This has helped countries purchase vaccines based on national plans when they need them, sustaining successful vaccine-preventable diseases programs and securing favorable bulk-purchase prices for epidemic and pandemic responses. The revolving fund provides countries with the option of either purchasing vaccines directly on submitting an order or utilizing 60-day interest-free financing with the expectation that they will mobilize the resources required to reimburse the fund during that period or accumulate interest. The default rate since inception of the revolving fund has been less than 10%. For each dose of vaccine sold through the revolving fund, countries pay an additional 4.25% fee to cover administrative costs (1.75%) and contribute to a capital fund (2.5%) that provides countries with credit for vaccine purchase if needed. In 2022, the revolving fund provided more than 235 million doses of vaccine to 41 countries, with more than 1,000 nationally programmed vaccine shipments through the revolving fund. During the COVID-19 pandemic, the revolving fund was the source of COVID-19 vaccine purchase for many countries in this region. The main complaint levelled against the revolving fund comes from industry, which has said that it constrains their profitability in countries that choose not to have bilateral price negotiations.

Sources: Hui Yang, The Global Fund. 2025. Symposium on Multilateral Financing for Pandemic Preparedness. INSPIRE Health Forum. Manila; and Santiago Cornejo, PAHO Revolving Fund. 2025. Symposium on Multilateral Financing for Pandemic Preparedness. INSPIRE Health Forum. Manila.

The central challenge lies in addressing incentive compatibility constraints: individual countries must perceive benefits that they would otherwise not realize by procuring health products independently (e.g., lower prices, better delivery terms, reliable supplies).[55] This alignment is not always straightforward, particularly across a wide range of products with varying market dynamics. A pragmatic entry point is to start with a small subset of products where national procurement volumes are low. In such cases, pooling demand is more likely to generate visible and immediate benefits, thereby guaranteeing incentive compatibility and strengthening trust in the mechanism. Importantly, VTD-like products that also have routine uses, such as monoclonal antibodies, antivirals, or reserve antibiotics, offer a practical opportunity. Focusing on these products keeps collaborative procurement squarely within the VTD and pandemic preparedness agenda, while addressing real needs faced by health systems today. This helps build political and institutional support for collaborative mechanisms that can be built on.

▶ Ensuring last-mile service delivery

Extending formal health care into communities. Extending the formal health care system into communities can take many forms, and lessons can be drawn from the successes and challenges of the COVID-19 pandemic. Many countries established new sites for COVID-19 testing and delivery of vaccines and other medical commodities. Generally, these were temporary and were limited by the lack of qualified personnel to take specimens and perform laboratory tests. Brazil scaled up testing by passing legislation to allow its 94,000 pharmacies to offer COVID-19 testing. This dramatically increased access to diagnostics, and pharmacists welcomed the added responsibilities in delivering point-of-care testing for COVID-19 and chronic disease management, as well as administering COVID-19 vaccines.[56] In addition, the enlistment of pharmacists led to the discovery of millions of people who only ever used pharmacies and never accessed formal health facilities, calling attention to persistent health system challenges.

55 N. Privett and P. Yadav. 2015. *Analysis of the Procurement and Pricing Architecture for Vaccines.* Working Paper. NYU Wagner.

56 C. Piquer-Martinez et al. 2022. Integration of Community Pharmacy in Primary Health Care: The Challenge. *Research in Social and Administrative Pharmacy*. 18 (8). pp. 3444–3447.

CHAPTER 4

An Investment Road Map for More Equitable, Effective, and Agile Pandemic Solutions

There is no instant solution: long-term health system resilience in Asia and the Pacific can only be achieved through sustained attention and action.

A Call to Action

COVID-19 was a stress test for health, economic, and governance systems worldwide, and its lessons remain pressing. Unpreparedness carries cascading consequences: collapsing health services, reversing development gains, and destabilizing economies. The magnitude of global losses, measured in trillions of dollars and millions of lives, demonstrated that preparedness is not a discretionary expense but a foundation of macroeconomic stability. Countries that invested early in surveillance, resilient systems, and inclusive access to health care managed to contain shocks and recover faster, proving that health security and economic security are inseparable.

For Asia and the Pacific, the path forward lies in transforming vulnerability into long-term resilience. Pandemic readiness must be a permanent consideration and embedded into fiscal and development planning, not just an emergency measure. The region's diverse economies can draw on collective strengths in manufacturing capacity, technological innovation, and regional cooperation. International financial institutions can help align public investment with global standards and private capital.

The coming decade presents a narrow but decisive window to consolidate these gains. Climate change, urbanization, and ecological disruption are intensifying the risk of new zoonotic spillovers. The chance that a COVID-19-like or worse pandemic might occur over the next 25 years has been estimated at around 50%.[57] Meeting this challenge demands a shift from episodic response to continuous readiness, from piecemeal and isolated health interventions to integrated systems that blend considerations for health, the environment, and economies. Strengthening regional solidarity, transparency, and mutual accountability will be vital in ensuring that no country is left exposed when the next threat emerges. By treating health resilience as a public good, the region can turn its experience of crisis into a model of sustained, inclusive security.

An Investment Road Map

How can we transform these lessons into a cohesive, actionable pandemic prevention, preparedness, and response investment agenda?

We propose four pillars to reify an equitable, effective and agile pandemic prevention, preparedness, and response (PPPR) system across all of Asia and the Pacific (Figure 9):

PILLAR 1 **Strategy—increase the strategic focus on PPPR, UHC, and health resilience**

- Governments, multilateral institutions, and other partners should consider PPPR to be a public good and increase

[57] S. Sharma et al., eds. 2026. *Investing in Pandemic Prevention, Preparedness, and Response*. Disease Control Priorities, 4th ed., Vol. 2. World Bank.

investments in resilient health systems and UHC—strengthening health infrastructure, health access, diagnostic capabilities, and research and surveillance systems. Multilateral development banks (MDBs), such as ADB, are uniquely positioned to facilitate regional cooperation—enhancing regional and cross-border surveillance and data sharing, and promoting the One Health approach. Strategic targeting of hot spots with the highest risk of spillovers should be prioritized, and efforts to prevent disease emergence intensified. Crucially, pandemics should also be recognized as national and international security threats and embedded within defense and security policies, plans, and budgets accordingly.

PILLAR 2 Finance—improve the efficiency and impact of PPPR investments

- Governments should increase budget allocations for PPPR, mobilize domestic resources, track spending, and accelerate the uptake of PPPR-relevant public financial management (PFM) reforms. MDBs have ready instruments to support the PFM-strengthening agenda (e.g., policy-based lending, technical assistance). At the same time, external aid should be integrated into national health sector plans, budget cycles, and PFM systems to strengthen accountability, efficiency, and coherence of investments. MDBs can ensure adequate and sustainable financing for pandemics by establishing day-zero financing: a prearranged, timely surge response credit line. In addition, MDBs can mainstream PPPR investments by integrating preparedness metrics into operations; aligning loans with results-based triggers linked to surveillance, emergency response, and service continuity; and leveraging private capital through blended instruments that de-risk investment in health infrastructure and supply chains. Embracing the concept of additionality, MDBs should leverage lending with the grants of the Pandemic Fund and philanthropy.

PILLAR 3 Governance—embrace bold, sustained governance action at multiple levels

- Multilateral institutions and other partners should prioritize and expand regional harmonization and regionally coordinated national plans and policies. This includes scaling-up capacity for data sharing and regional collaboration on vaccines, therapeutics, and diagnostics (VTDs). ADB's Greater Mekong and Central Asia Regional Economic Cooperation subregions offer existing models of collaboration, harmonization, and data-sharing for health. To strengthen global governance, donors, international organizations, and regional entities should align mandates, notably through the new Coordinating Financial Mechanism to be established under the Pandemic Agreement. Governments should establish legal and institutional frameworks for pandemic response before the next crisis strikes, ensuring synergies between community-led and government-led efforts, particularly around social protection, risk communication, community engagement, and cross-sector coordination.

PILLAR 4 Medical countermeasure security—invest in a regional ecosystem for the development, manufacturing, and regulation of VTDs and other pandemic tools

- Governments, multilateral institutions, and other partners should invest in regional manufacturing of vaccines for priority pathogens and other underinvested products (e.g., diagnostics, personal protective equipment). Investments in R&D are critical to sustain innovation pipelines, as are efforts to strengthen national regulatory authorities in LMICs.

MDBs should establish regional mechanisms for collaborative procurement and equitable distribution of vaccines, retooling procurement models to share risk with suppliers and incentivize supplier readiness. Collaborating with partners such as CEPI to design analytics for at-risk procurement portfolios, and piloting regional or subregional collaborative procurement mechanisms for routine medicines can yield substantial benefits during emergencies—ensuring decisions can be made with speed, reducing fragmentation and market power asymmetries, and promoting equity.

Figure 9: An Investment Road Map for More Equitable, Effective, and Agile Pandemic Solutions

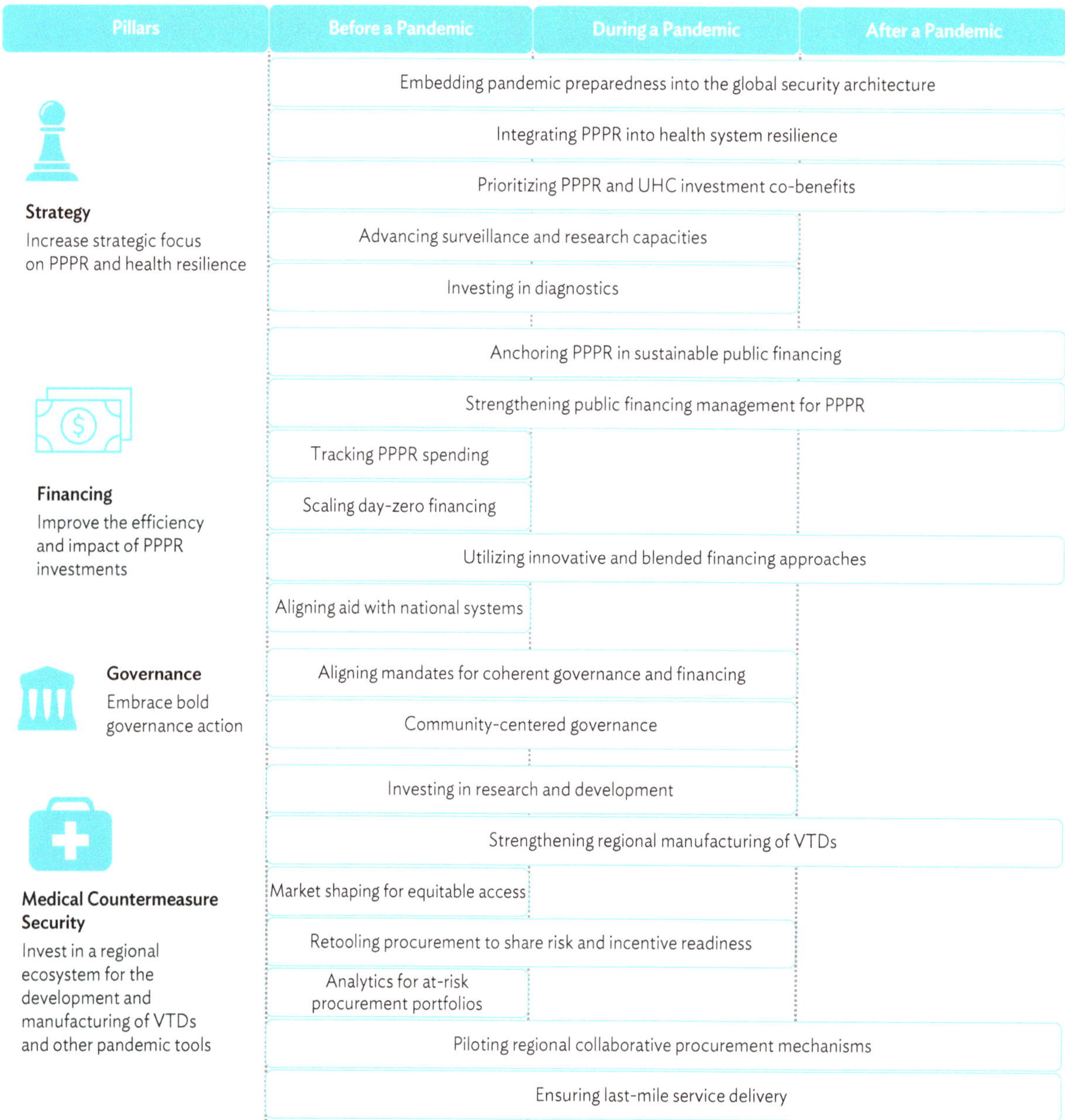

PPPR = pandemic prevention, preparedness, and response; UHC = universal health coverage; VTDs = vaccines, therapeutics, and diagnostics.

Source: Asian Development Bank.

www.ingramcontent.com/pod-product-compliance
Lightning Source LLC
Chambersburg PA
CBHW041759220926
51847CB00014B/259